Managing Urinary Incontinence in the Elderly

John F. Schnelle, PhD is Associate Director, Borun Center for Gerontological Research and Professor in Residence, Multicampus Division of Geriatric Medicine and Gerontology, School of Medicine, University of California, Los Angeles. He is renowned for his role as principal investigator on several major clinical trial intervention grants designed to improve care and management in nursing homes, and has received awards for his outstanding contributions to behavior therapy. Among his most notable contributions is his innovative work in incontinence care. Dr. Schnelle has published extensively in the areas of quality control in institutional settings and quality-of-life issues in the frail elderly, with over 60 publications in professional books and journals. He currently serves on the Board of Editors of *The Journal of Organizational Behavior Management.*

Managing Urinary Incontinence in the Elderly

John F. Schnelle, PhD

Springer Publishing Company
New York

Springer Publishing Company, Inc.
536 Broadway
New York, NY 10012-3955

90 91 92 93 94 95 / 5 4 3 2 1

Library of Congress Cataloging-in-Publication Data

Schnelle, John F.
Managing urinary incontinence in the elderly / John F. Schnelle.
p. cm.
Includes bibliographical references and index.
ISBN 0-8261-7360-8
1. Urinary incontinence—Patients—Rehabilitation. 2. Urinary incontinence—Nursing. 3. Nursing home care. 4. Aged—Rehabilitation. I. Title.
[DNLM: 1. Aged. 2. Urinary Incontinence—nursing.
3. Urinary
Incontinence—rehabilitation. WJ 146 S359m]
RC921.I5S48 1991
362.1'9897662—dc20
DNLM/DLC
for Library of Congress 90-10430
CIP

Printed in the United States of America

To Ruth Catherine, with thanks

CONTENTS

LIST OF FIGURES

PREFACE

Urinary incontinence may be viewed as an unnecessarily serious problem among many elderly people, because recent research has shown that incontinence can be effectively treated and managed. The purpose of this volume is to avoid the unnecessary predicament of urinary incontinence. Nursing home professionals and home care providers can significantly reduce incontinence problems in even the most debilitated elderly by following the procedures outlined in the following chapters. While obviously relevant to an important clinical problem, the patient care and staff-management model illustrated herein for the problem of incontinence may be applied to other areas of patient care.

It is an unfortunate truth that elderly neglect occurs most frequently with people who are the most debilitated. The frail elderly need the most assistance with basic life needs; neglect occurs when care providers are not consistently attentive. The present book is designed to describe quality control and management procedures that increase the probability of consistent incontinence care. The same techniques can also be used to assure consistent care in regard to eating, exercise, and a variety of other important care areas.

The management technology described in Chapters 4, 5, and 6 borrows heavily from the staff management and quality-control measures used in business settings to improve the quality of products and services. These techniques are generally accepted and used by both national and international businesses. This volume describes one of the first examples of how this powerful quality-control technology can be used to facilitate an important patient outcome.

Computer software to facilitate all computations relevant to patient assessment (Chapter 4) and quality control (Chapter 6) is available by contacting the author at UCLA School of Medicine, Borun Center for Gerontological Research, Los Angeles, California.

ACKNOWLEDGMENTS

The quality-control technology used to maintan consistent incontinence care has been influenced by the work of Edward Demming. The early work of Dr. Todd Risely and Nathan Azrin also provided examples of how behavioral research should be organized and conducted. Dr. Carl Adams motivated much of the early incontinence work that lead to this research. The National Health Corporation has provided many excellent nursing facility test sites. Dan Newman, Marilyn White, Ann Haynes and many other research associates were instrumental in completing this research.

The research that has formed the basis for this book was supported by the National Institute on Aging and the Division of Nursing Research. Dr. Marcia Ory has been a very supportive project officer and friend.

Chapter 1

THE PROBLEM OF URINARY INCONTINENCE

What to learn from this chapter:

1. **How prevalent urinary incontinence is in elderly patients.**
2. **What can be done about urinary incontinence.**
3. **The difference between nursing management and treatment of urinary incontinence.**
4. **Why so many incontinent people are in nursing homes.**
5. **How this book can help with elderly people who live at home.**
6. **The different types of incontinence.**
7. **Who can benefit from incontinence training.**

Urinary incontinence occurs when people involuntarily leak or lose urine. In most nursing home patients, bowel incontinence, or loss of stool, accompanies urinary incontinence.

Many people think incontinence is a normal part of aging and that it results from severe illness or strokes. It is also widely believed that little can be done about this problem. These beliefs are dangerous. They prevent nurse's aides and other caregivers from attempting to solve or alleviate incontinence problems. Unfortunately, these beliefs find partial basis in fact. Incontinence is more likely to occur in older people. Aging, as well as many of the health problems that affect older people often increases the risk of incontinence. Increased occurrence, however, does not mean that caregivers should give up and do nothing. It may be more difficult for elderly people to stay continent, but it certainly is not impossible.

Older people and their caregivers just have to work harder to minimize incontinence, and this book demonstrates how it can be done. The theme that older people must compensate for problems that make staying continent more difficult is emphasized repeatedly throughout. The following case study illustrates this theme.

CASE OF MRS. X

Mrs. X was a 92-year-old nursing home patient who could not hear well and who could walk only with assistance from other people. Her hearing problem made it difficult to talk with her. She had lived in the nursing home for 2 years after being admitted from the hospital where she was treated for a broken hip. She had been catheterized in the hospital and continued to be catheterized for 1 month after admission to the nursing home. When the catheter was removed, she could feel bladder pressure only for a few minutes before voiding. The interval between feeling the sensation to void and voiding was so short that she did not have time to ask for toileting assistance. In addition, for several weeks after the catheter was removed, she had to void 12 to 15 times per day. Mrs. X was incontinent, and she found incontinence both embarrassing and uncomfortable. The nursing staff did not seem concerned about the problem and changed Mrs. X along with her roommate, who was also incontinent. Because Mrs. X remained in considerable pain from the hip fracture, it was painful for her to move, and she did not make a point of asking for toileting assistance.

Mrs. X gradually enjoyed partial recovery from the hip fracture. She no longer suffered severe pain and could sit in a chair comfortably for 4 to 6 hours at a time. She had been incontinent for 4 months at this point and no longer attached significance to the problem. Most other patients in the nursing home were incontinent, and the staff accepted the condition as a normal part of their care routines. At this point, Mrs. X had been wet for so long that she no longer could tell whether she was wet or dry. In short, she adapted to the condition and accepted it as a normal part of her life. She did not request toileting assistance or complain about being wet, and the nursing staff assumed that Mrs. X accepted her condition and that her needs were being met.

A rehabilitative nurse decided to assess Mrs. X for her incontinence problem. During the first day of assessment, Mrs. X was checked every hour for wetness and was asked simple questions such as "Are you wet?" or "Are you dry?" Mrs. X attempted to answer the questions even though she was not sure about the answers. The staff told her whether she was correct when she answered the questions and encouraged her to try to feel whether she was wet or dry. The staff found her answers correct about 67% of the time.

Mrs. X was wet six different times between 7:00 A.M. and 7:00 P.M. on the first assessment day. This represents a very high voiding frequency, but the staff recognized one good sign. On one occasion she had a 200-cc void. This large void indicated that Mrs. X's bladder was still able to hold a relatively large volume of urine. If Mrs. X could hold 200 cc of urine, she should be able to wait at least 2 hours between toiletings without becoming wet. Because Mrs. X attempted to answer questions about whether she was wet or dry and because of the one high voiding volume, the rehabilitative nurse carried Mrs. X into a second assessment day. During the second assessment day, Mrs. X was checked every hour for wetness and was asked if she was wet or dry. In addition, she was now asked if she would try to use the toilet. Staff members were pleasant but persuasive. They asked Mrs. X if she would really "try" to use the toilet. If she said no the first time, she was prompted to toilet. They then asked again and talked to her more about the problem before they left. When she did try to use the toilet, the staff reacted enthusiastically and praised her efforts.

Mrs. X said she wanted to use the toilet and used it successfully three times during the second assessment day. More important, she was incontinent only twice that day, as opposed to six times the day before, when she did not try to toilet. The two incontinence accidents she had were small. Thus, Mrs. X was not as wet nor as frequently wet as previously. This response convinced the rehabilitative nurse to keep Mrs. X on a 1-hour toileting schedule for 3 more days. She continued to do well and gradually developed more sensation as to whether she was wet or dry.

Because the staff seemed to care so much, Mrs. X would ask for toileting assistance even before a staff member prompted her. She soon discovered that she would have to use the toilet about four times in an 8-hour period if she was to succeed in holding her urine between toiletings. She still did not feel a strong sensation to void, and what little sensation she had occurred only a few minutes before voiding. The only thing she could do was void frequently, even when she did not feel she had to. After 1 week, the staff nurse checked Mrs. X only every 2 hours and prompted her to toilet. She continued to do well and continued to try to toilet every 2 hours. She was still wet occasionally, but it was usually a small leakage that occurred about once a day. Most typically, Mrs. X would have a small leakage after she coughed or was moved to a standing position by a nurse's aide.

In short, Mrs. X had to go to the bathroom more often than when she was 50, and she was still wet occasionally. Her incontinence improved, however, and she remained dry most of the time. She was taught a new toileting strategy by the nursing staff. She had to do things differently from when she was young because of her health problems, but Mrs. X had successfully compensated for the problems.

NURSING MANAGEMENT VERSUS MEDICAL TREATMENT

This book emphasizes a nursing management approach to urinary incontinence. This approach differs from medical treatment, which involves drugs or surgery. The nursing management approach teaches people behaviors that can reduce and in some cases reverse severe urinary incontinence. Expensive equipment and specialized professional services are not necessary to implement the nursing management strategy. The procedures described here are relatively simple and can be used with extremely ill or frail patients. Procedures described in this book therefore prove useful in all nursing homes and in many home-care settings. If implemented correctly, these procedures improve incontinence symptoms in about 50% to 70% of all patients. Some patients will even become totally continent. These improvements occur without exposing patients to the risks and problems associated with surgery or medication.

Despite the advantages and effectiveness of nursing management procedures, incontinent patients should be assessed by a physician. If a patient is relatively strong, surgery will help some types of incontinence. It is less certain, but possible, that some drugs may also prove beneficial. Note, however, that even if clients pursue medical intervention, the nursing procedures described in this book provide useful supplements to medical treatment. In the case of patients who cannot toilet independently, the procedures described in this book must be implemented if medical treatment is to succeed.

There is little to lose and much to gain by initiating the nursing management approach. You will find that many incontinence accidents experienced by patients reflect a failure to compensate for problems that make accidents likely. As in the case study, some elderly people may have to be taught to go to the bathroom more frequently and at times when they do not feel a strong bladder pressure. Such frequent toileting will reduce bladder pressure and decrease the number of times accidents occur. Other patients may not be able to get to a toilet quickly or, in the case of nursing home patients, may not be able to toilet independently at all. These patients need consistent toileting assistance. Such regular assistance, if given correctly, will significantly improve incontinence in most patients. The problem is how to manage nurse's aides and other caregivers so that such assistance is provided continuously. The system devised to solve this nursing management problem is described in this book.

NURSING HOME CARE

There are about 1.5 million nursing home patients, and at least half suffer from urinary incontinence (Ouslander, Kane, & Abrass, 1982). Many of these same patients also experience bowel, or fecal, incontinence (Ouslander et al., 1982). Health costs of nursing home incontinence are high. Incontinence has been associated with skin lesions, depression, and urinary tract infection. Labor and laundry costs involved in changing patients and additional costs of treating patients for health problems associated with incontinence have been estimated in excess of $1.5 billion per year (Ouslander & Kane, 1984).

Incontinence remains prevalent in nursing homes because so many incontinent patients are immobile or otherwise unable to utilize a toileting receptacle independently. In fact, about 86% of nursing home patients are not capable of independent toileting (Schnelle, Sowell, Traughber, & Hu, 1988). In addition, many patients suffer from memory, attention, or motivational problems, which lower the chance that patients will ask for toileting assistance before incontinence occurs.

Combined, these problems can mean only one thing if incontinence in nursing home patients is to be improved or even well managed. Nursing staff must contact patients on a consistent basis and persuasively offer toileting assistance to those capable of using a toilet. Unfortunately, many nursing homes cannot ensure consistent patient–staff contact. Staff shortages, training problems, and poor personnel management all contribute to this problem.

When nursing home incontinence care is poor due to inconsistent staff performance, other patient-care areas tend also to be poor. A basic premise underlying most patient care in nursing homes is that the staff maintain regular contact with patients. Such consistent contact is required to prevent skin breakdown and falls, to remove restraints, or to offer water. If the nursing staff do a poor job of toileting patients and otherwise keeping patients dry, they may also do a poor job in other patient-care areas. In fact, survey teams responsible for evaluating nursing home care frequently measure how many patients are wet. They consider these measures good indicators of overall patient-care quality.

In general, incontinence among nursing home patients can improve dramatically if the staff consistently contact patients on a 2-hour schedule and offer toileting assistance in the correct way. Implementing a successful toileting program increases the probability that overall patient care will also improve. How nurse managers can design, implement, and manage a successful incontinence program is discussed throughout this book.

HOME CARE

Many elderly people with incontinence problems live at home, either alone or with assistance from a home health care provider. It is estimated that 15% to 30% of elderly people who live at home suffer from urinary incontinence (Diokno, Brock, Brown, & Herzog, 1986).

In general, elderly persons who live at home are not as ill or as debilitated as are nursing home patients. In fact, the primary concern of elderly persons living at home is to prevent further health deterioration so that nursing home placement will not be necessary. Several writers identify urinary incontinence as one of the primary reasons that families and patients seek nursing home care (Palmer, 1988). Treating and reducing the severity of urinary incontinence symptoms is one way to prevent the need for nursing home placement.

Many of the same management principles that work with nursing home patients also work well with nonambulatory elderly persons who live at home. The fact remains that incontinence severity is exaggerated by a failure to compensate for factors that make the problem worse. Elderly persons living at home can be taught to identify and act on these factors. In so doing, they reduce many accidents. Procedures the elderly and their caregivers can use to better manage incontinence in the home are the major focus of Chapter 8.

TYPES OF INCONTINENCE

Incontinence problems can be categorized into several major groups. Correct diagnosis or labeling of incontinence is important for good medical treatment. Some of the more common types of incontinence can be recognized by the symptoms.

Stress incontinence, for example, can be recognized when small amounts of urine are leaked after a cough or when exercising or laughing. Coughing increases abdominal pressure and places more pressure on the bladder. Many people have weakened musculature around the bladder outlet that prevents them from holding their urine in the presence of such pressure. An operation called bladder neck suspension is a commonly used medical procedure to treat stress incontinence (Resnick & Yalla, 1985).

Urge incontinence can be recognized when people cannot delay voiding long enough to reach the toilet after the urge to void is felt. In many cases people also feel they must go to the bathroom frequently. A high-frequency voiding rate would be more than 10 times per 24-hour period. Some diseases, such as strokes and parkinsonism, can lead to urge incontinence (Resnick & Yalla, 1985). There are some medications for urge incontinence problems, but behavioral management is probably the most commonly used treatment technique. Bladder drill or bladder retraining and even biofeedback training can be used with urge-incontinence problems. If a patient is capable of following instructions and does not show severe mental deficits, training procedures can be utilized successfully. Chapter 8 discusses how to implement these behavioral procedures.

Overflow incontinence occurs when the bladder cannot empty because of an obstruction in the voiding channel. This problem is most common in men who have enlarged prostate glands. It may also occur in diabetes, neuropathy, or spinal cord injury. Typically, overflow incontinence is treated with intermittent catheterization or surgical removal of the obstruction (Resnick & Yalla, 1985).

Functional incontinence occurs when people refuse to use the toilet either because of psychological problems or because limited mobility restricts their ability to get to a toilet. In addition, patients who suffer from Alzheimer's disease or organic brain disease may not remember how or when to use a toilet. Patients with functional incontinence usually do not have severe urological problems. There is no common medical treatment for this disorder. Behavioral programs that involve toileting patients on a scheduled basis are perhaps the most typical procedure used for this problem (Hadley, 1986).

WHO CAN BE MANAGED

It would be a mistake not to consider all patients with incontinence problems as potential candidates for one of the management approaches. For example, bed-bound nursing home patients who cannot even tell what day it is have responded to the nursing management procedures described in this book. These procedures have also been successful with each type of incontinence described in the preceding section.

Unfortunately, about 35% of all nursing home patients will never be able to toilet well enough to improve incontinence. It remains unclear how many elderly persons living at home would be unresponsive. Despite the fact that many incontinence problems will not improve with management or treatment, all persons should be assessed and at least considered for management. In most cases, a trial of at least one noninvasive treatment or management procedure is worthwhile, no matter how debilitated the patient appears. Many patients will not become completely continent, but they may at least become drier.

Assessing the incontinence problem may mean going to a physician, usually a urologist, and specifically asking for help for incontinence. Important assessment information can also be collected by nurses, other caregivers, and even patients themselves. This book outlines an inexpensive method for collecting and, more important, interpreting assessment information. This assessment information, collected over a 6-day period, will help identify patients who are excellent candidates for incontinence management. The information also can be used to design effective plans for containing incontinence in patients who are not good candidates for rehabilitation. Home-care providers who assist severely debilitated patients who cannot use the toilet can employ the same assessment and treatment procedures that are utilized by nursing home personnel.

The first seven chapters in this book describe how to assess, treat, and manage incontinence problems in the frail elderly who, because of physical and mental problems, cannot take care of their own needs. Patients may show any type of incontinence discussed in this chapter, but they are more likely to exhibit urge and functional incontinence problems. Chapter 8 describes various assessment and treatment procedures for elderly patients who have the physical or mental capacity to toilet independently. Most of these patients live at home instead of in nursing homes. Chapter 8 should be read by the patients themselves as well as by their home health care providers.

REFERENCES

Diokno, A. C., Brock, B. M., Brown, M. B., & Herzog, A. R. (1986). Prevalence of urinary incontinence and other urological symptoms in the non-institutionalized elderly. *Journal of Urology, 136*(5), 1022–1025.

Hadley, E. C. (1986). Bladder training and related therapies for urinary incontinence in older people. *Journal of the American Medical Association, 256*(3), 372–379.

Ouslander, J. G., & Kane, R. L. (1984). The costs of urinary incontinence in nursing homes. *Medical Care, 22,* 69–74.

Ouslander, J. G., Kane, R. L., & Abrass, I. B. (1982). Urinary incontinence in elderly nursing home patients. *Journal of the American Medical Association, 248,* 1194–1198.

Palmer, M. H. (1988). Incontinence: The magnitude of the problem. *Nursing Clinics of North America, 23*(11), 139–157.

Resnick, N. M., & Yalla, S. V. (1985). Management of urinary incontinence in the elderly. *New England Journal of Medicine, 313*(13), 800–805.

Schnelle, J. F., Sowell, V. A., Traughber, B., & Hu, T. W. (1988). A behavioral analysis of the labor cost of managing continence and incontinence in nursing home patients. *Journal of Organizational Behavior Management, 9*(2), 137–153.

Chapter 2

STARTING A PROGRAM

What to learn from this chapter:

1. **The federal standards for incontinence care.**
2. **The key points in a successful rehabilitation program.**
3. **How training and management interact in starting the incontinence program.**
4. **What common misconceptions aides and other caregivers share about incontinence rehabilitation.**
5. **How a supervisor should react to these misconceptions.**
6. **What physicians, family members, and patients should know about the program.**

Starting an incontinence program involves both training nursing staff and communicating key program points to physicians, patients, and family members. This chapter describes how such training and communication procedures can begin.

To understand the importance of the major rehabilitation program points it is useful to understand first the federal regulations relating to incontinence care in nursing homes. The rules are clearly written and are more specific than standards written in the past. Despite improved clarity, however, nurse managers will find that many of the guidelines remain open to interpretation. The guidelines outline basic principles for conducting incontinence care; the actual mechanics of implementing the rules are left to the ingenuity of nurse managers.

The most general incontinence care standard states that "residents with incontinence are provided with the care necessary to encourage continence including frequent toileting and opportunities for rehabilitative nursing." To implement this general standard, the guidelines articulate a series of more specific recommendations. These key rules are summarized as follows:

1. Recent admissions and newer incontinent patients should be assessed thoroughly for the cause of their incontinence; and, when appropriate, an intensive bowel and bladder program should be developed.
2. There should be a written care plan for all incontinent residents. For those on bowel and bladder retraining, progress notes should be written. The care plan should outline goals and specify toileting schedules.
3. There should be a chart in the resident's room on which the patient's response to the program is documented.
4. There should be evidence of follow-through in the implementation of the rehabilitation program.
5. For residents not on bowel and bladder retraining, there should be a care plan which addresses specific measures to manage incontinence. (American Health Care Association, 1987)

To summarize these rules, all patients should be assessed, individualized treatment or incontinence management strategies should be implemented, and quality assurance documentation data should be collected. This book deals specifically with implementation of these assessment, treatment, and quality assurance rules.

KEY REHABILITATION PROGRAM POINTS

Don't Toilet Everybody

Most nursing home programs make a major mistake in placing too many and the wrong type of patients on toileting schedules. About 25% to 35% of incontinent nursing home patients have difficulty in starting the voiding process. These patients can be placed on a toilet, but they will not be able to void. This toileting "dry run" is not only time-consuming but very frustrating to the staff. Placing even a few of these patients on a toileting program effectively reduces staff performance with all patients. Patients who can initiate voiding are not given the toileting assistance they need. In addition to staff motivation and lost time, placing unresponsive patients on a toileting schedule has serious implications for the nurse manager's ability to maintain quality control.

Selecting only patients who can respond is the first step in developing a successful incontinence rehabilitation program. This patient-selection process can be deceptive. Patients who are very verbal may have urological problems that make them poor candidates for a toileting program. Alternatively, barely responsive patients, who score 0 on mental status exams, have been able to respond well. In other words, you cannot correctly select patients just by talking to them or by picking the most healthy-looking.

Fortunately, an assessment system has been developed that allows nurse managers to select "responsive" patients. This assessment process can be implemented easily within a 1-to-6-day period by trained nurse's aides. Chapter 4 describes this process and teaches supervisors to utilize assessment data to make treatment decisions.

Don't Automatically Toilet: Talk

The most difficult obstacle to implementing a toileting program is getting the staff in consistent contact with patients. Once in contact with patients, the staff must learn to communicate with them in a meaningful and humane manner. Many nurse's aides will perform patient-care routines without talking to patients. Patients quickly become passive and overly dependent under these conditions.

If this noncommunicative style is carried over to a toileting program, staff will often automatically toilet a patient without first talking about the toileting process. This automatic, "scheduled" toileting procedure has several drawbacks. First, an opportunity is lost to talk to patients about a subject they can respond to no matter how disoriented they may be. Patients may not know what day it is, but they may be able to tell you whether they are wet or dry. Teaching staff to ask a patient such simple questions as "Are you wet?" or "Are you dry?" is a good start in an overall patient-orientation program. Most important, it will take staff no more time to talk to the patient about toileting than it will simply to toilet automatically.

Second, toileting patients without talking to them and preparing them for the toileting event is inefficient. Toileting a patient who does not need or want to be toileted will prove frustrating to the patient and will result in more dry runs. A dry run occurs when a patient tries to use a toilet but cannot initiate voiding. A prompted-voiding procedure, which includes a simple communication protocol that nurses can use before toileting a patient, is described in Chapter 3.

Active Chart Recording

All professional rehabilitation programs require that patient progress be monitored and documented. In the case of incontinence rehabilitation, the person providing incontinence care must routinely record data concerning the patient's incontinence status and toileting behavior. Typically, a nursing home will hang a chart in the patient's room and rely exclusively on nurse's aides to record incontinence data.

Unfortunately, nurse's aides often do not record information accurately with such a passive approach. Frequently, they do not record information during the shift at all. When reminded at the end of the shift, the aide will often complete the chart from memory, which increases the chance for inaccuracy. A recording system must be devised to minimize such problems if documentation is to be anything but a paper game. The system described in this book addresses this problem by emphasizing a more active recording approach.

This system works because it differs in two major areas from normal recording procedures. First, floor nurses and supervisors are responsible for entering information on the chart at least once per day. Thus, both nurse's aides and their supervisors actually use the toileting chart. Supervisors enter information concerning the patient's wet or dry status, as well as information about how well aides are managing the toileting schedule. This system emphasizes to nurse's aides the importance of documentation procedures because supervisors show that they are paying attention to the information recorded.

Second, toileting documentation sheets are placed on clipboards, and nurse's aides are instructed to return the clipboards to the nurses' station at the end of each shift. Nurse's aides on the following shift are requested to take the clipboards to the patients' rooms at the beginning of their shift. This procedure serves several major purposes. It reminds the staff which patients are on the program by requiring an overt behavioral act: transporting the clipboards. It also brings the aide in contact with the patient at two critical times: at the beginning and the end of each shift. Finally, it gives supervisors an opportunity to screen all of the charts quickly while they are together at the nurses' station. How this documentation system should be implemented is described in Chapter 5.

Quality Control

Nurses aides are charged with major responsibility for incontinence care and aides will perform best if they receive ongoing support from supervisors. Training, without such follow-up supervision, will not be effective and no incontinence program will succeed without a quality control program. Quality control must come from directors of nurses and their professional nurse assistants.

This fact should not be surprising. There are few work situations in which hourly workers are hired to perform important job tasks without quality control. Unfortunately, health care falls behind manufacturing in its ability to develop and implement good quality-control systems. Several major steps comprise any quality-control process:

1. Specific criteria and expected standards of job performance must be set.
2. There must be procedures for collecting accurate information about the quality of current job performance.
3. There must be a way to compare current work performance with expected performance standards.
4. There should be a means of identifying reasons for differences between desired levels of performance and actual performance.
5. There should be a means for collecting information regarding

improvements in work performance that occur when changes are made.

6. The quality-control system should be ongoing and dynamic. It should permit the constant interaction of all of the previous steps.

These basic principles of quality control have been translated into a system of measures and procedures that help maintain the excellence of incontinence rehabilitation programming. This book shows how to set performance standards that specify how "dry" patients should be if staff are performing well-defined patient-care routines. Second, a monitoring system is described that allows nurse managers to collect information about how well aides are keeping patients dry. Third, control charts are presented that permit the comparison of daily incontinence care to standards that have been set. In cases where discrepancies occur between daily performance and expected performance, procedures have been instituted to correct the problem. Finally, the entire system is designed to be ongoing and to prevent problems. The goal is not to detect poor performance after it occurs but to monitor work performance continuously.

In short, the product of nursing homes is patient care, and the performance of nurse's aides relates directly to this product. Nurse's aides' performance must be monitored and measured closely if patient care is to reach a consistently high quality. A quality-control system that accomplishes these objectives is described in Chapter 6.

TRAINING AND MANAGEMENT

Nurse's Aides and Floor Nurses

There are three major groups of people involved in implementing successful nursing home incontinence programs: nurse's aides, floor nurses, and supervisory nurses responsible for overall care in the facility. The following chapters define the specific incontinence-program responsibilities of each of these groups. Nurse's aides have the most direct responsibility and engage in the most "hands on" patient care. These aides are trained in two ways: in-service classroom training and on-the-job floor training. This book emphasizes an approach that limits in-service training sessions for nurse's aides. Two classroom sessions, approximately 20 to 25 minutes each, are all that is required.

This approach emphasizes floor training for two major reasons. First, it is difficult to get floor nurses and aides to change their patient-care behavior based on what they learn in the classroom. It is difficult for any occupational group to translate classroom information to job performance. Second, major incontinence activities required of aides and floor nurses are not complicated. In fact, they are not much different from current duties. In other words, managing aide behavior is more vital than training for new behavior.

In recognition of this fact, primary emphasis focuses on floor training and follow-up quality-control supervision. The few in-service sessions that should be held are not designed to communicate specific job performance requirements. The objectives of such training sessions are (a) to identify and correct misconceptions about incontinence care in the elderly, (b) to communicate to floor aides and nurses that good patient care can make a difference, (c) to identify and address common resistances to rehabilitation programs, and (d) to communicate strong supervisory support for the program.

These objectives can best be accomplished if nurse's aides and supervisors are given a brief pretest before the in-service training session. A discussion of aides' answers to the pretest provides a basis for a more personalized and interesting training session. The major questions that should be on this test are listed in Figure 2.1.

These questions address two common attitudes that nurse's aides often evidence about incontinence, which, if allowed to go unchallenged, undermine the effectiveness of rehabilitation programs. These two attitudes can be summarized as follows: "Incontinence is not an important problem to the patient" and "The nurse's aide can't do anything about it."

"Incontinence Is Not Important"

The first attitude is common among long-term-care workers for several reasons. One is that the frail elderly suffer many problems

1. Incontinence is not one of the more serious problems among nursing home patients? True____ False____
2. Incontinence cannot be changed in most nursing home patients because of medical problems. True____ False____
3. There is nothing nurses or aides can do to improve incontinence in most patients. True____ False____
4. Taking care of incontinent patients takes a lot more time than if a patient is continent. True____ False____
5. There is no real need to toilet most incontinent patients. They can't use it. True____ False____
6. A good requirement is that patients be checked for incontinence every 2 hours. True____ False____
7. I don't have time to toilet patients every 2 hours. True____ False____
8. There is no need to talk to patients about toileting before you toilet them. True____ False____
9. If patients do not ask for assistance, they don't care about incontinence. True____ False____

FIGURE 2.1 Nurse's aide test.

far more life-threatening and debilitative than incontinence. This point should be addressed by communicating to nurse's aides that more serious health problems are generally less reversible than incontinence. Thus, incontinence may not be one of the most severe problems experienced by frail patients, but it is a treatable problem. Good nursing care may not allow many stroke patients to walk again, but good nursing care can make a patient more continent. Care providers must understand that there is a strong base of scientific evidence that proves incontinence can be changed. Producing such incontinence improvements is a sign of good nursing care.

Misconceptions concerning the importance of incontinence also exist because of the passivity of many elderly patients themselves. Most nursing home patients will not ask for toileting assistance prior to voiding. Furthermore, patients who have experienced the problem for a number of years may not show gratitude when the staff changes or toilets them. Lack of patient reaction creates the impression among caregivers that incontinence is of little consequence to the patient.

The caregiver must understand that passive acceptance of incontinence is part of the overall dependency that characterizes many of the frail elderly. Furthermore, this acceptance, or dependency, is created at least in part by caregivers, who often communicate that such dependency is expected, thus creating a dependency cycle. The caregiver communicates to the elderly patient that it is acceptable to be wet, and the patient responds with a lack of concern. Because little concern is shown, the caregiver assumes that the elderly do not care about the problem. This dependency cycle, as it relates to incontinence, can be broken only if aides communicate to patients that it does make a difference if they are wet. If the caregiver shows concern, elderly patients also show more interest in their incontinence. This process must start with the nurse's aide or caregiver. The elderly must be taught to care about their basic bodily functions again. It is an unhealthy and unprofessional nursing service that does not encourage patients' concern.

"Can't Do Anything about It"

In addition to the attitude that incontinence is unimportant, many aides also believe they can have little impact on the problem. A typical aide response to a new incontinence program is "I don't have time."

In truth, aides may not have time if they continue old work habits. The nature of the incontinence program is to teach nurse's aides more efficient work habits. It has been proved that nursing homes with patient–staff ratios of 12 to 1 on the 7:00 A.M. to 3:00 P.M. shift and 18 to 1 on the evening shift can implement the procedures described in this book. Nurse managers must communicate to aides that they will have time if they work smarter, not harder.

Tasks required of aides are tasks they are supposed to perform already. They should be in contact with the patient every 2 hours, with the first contact occuring during the first hour of the shift. If the typical aide cares for five incontinent patients, two of these patients will likely be on the toileting program. This effort will require approximately 10 minutes every 2 hours. The other three patients must be changed on a timely basis. This task will require approximately 15 minutes every 2 hours. Aides do have time to perform this required, basic incontinence care.

Unfortunately, aides will not save a great amount of time by toileting patients instead of changing them. Helping a dependent patient use a toilet or bedpan remains just as time-consuming as changing the patient. However, toileting patients is simply good patient care. Changing patients who could be dry if toileted is bad patient care. This difference between good and bad care must be made clear.

Nursing assistants should be taught to schedule their time differently. Many technicians develop rigidly fixed work habits. For example, you may often hear "We can't toilet patients because we have to get the trays out or the food will get cold" or "We have to bathe between 9 A.M. and 11 A.M. and we can't toilet." The point must be made that they can do both. If aides spend 10 minutes with two toileting patients at the beginning of the 7:00 A.M. shift, they will not have to spend time again with those patients until 9:00 A.M. If they check with the patient at 9:00 A.M., they will not have to check again until 11:00 A.M. Such a schedule may be different, but it is not impossible given job demands. A good nurse manager will quickly dispell the notion that patients cannot be toileted because of time limitations.

Director of Nurses and Assistants

The most critical person in the implementation of a successful incontinence rehabilitation program is the director of nurses and her or his assistants. Professional supervisory nurses must assume direct responsibility during the first weeks of the program. Specifically, a quality assurance nurse must do quality-control checks at least once per day for the first 4 weeks. Information collected from these checks is given directly to floor supervisors, who then provide the information to the aides.

These quality-control checks by the director of nurses take approximately 15 to 20 minutes per day and serve several critical purposes. First, they communicate to floor nurses that the program is important. In so doing, they address many of the misconceptions described in the preceding section concerning the unimportance of incontinence. Second, they enable a supervisory nurse to collect specific and interpretable information about how correctly aides are checking patients and providing toileting assistance. This supervisory ability to evaluate performance will influence nurse's aides' work habits even if nothing else is done.

The quality-control system is designed so that a quality assurance nurse makes frequent checks at the beginning of the program. There is increased likelihood that aides will exhibit acceptable job performance at the beginning of the program and during times when the quality assurance nurse is most visible. These initial frequent checks therefore increase the probability that the majority of feedback is positive. Thus, initially, the quality-control system emphasizes positive reinforcement to aides.

In summary, the quality assurance nurse or his or her assistant assumes the role of motivator or quality control engineer for the incontinence program. This role is made more critical because of the history of failed rehabilitation programs in many nursing homes. Professional nurses are essential to breaking this pattern of failure by producing a successful program.

Physicians, Patients, and Families

Physicians, patients, and families play an important role in developing a good rehabilitation program. If these groups are excluded from the rehabilitation process, this role can prove adversarial instead of facilitative.

Federal regulations specify that patients should be informed about rehabilitation programs, and many nursing facilities require a physician's approval for patient participation. In addressing these issues, the nursing home should seize a public relations opportunity and communicate to all critical parties that the nursing home offers a "state of the art" incontinence rehabilitation service.

The following points should be communicated clearly to families, physicians, and patients, either in writing or personally. It must be clear that the nursing home has a responsibility to manage incontinence and treat it. This responsibility requires that all incontinent patients be assessed. Assessment procedures are noninvasive and pose no risk to the patient. The major risk to the patient occurs when procedures are not implemented properly.

All relevant parties must understand that incontinence is not a natural condition and will not be accepted if it can be treated. A sign of good patient care is that patients are kept as dry as possible given the limitations of their condition. Thus, the nursing home has the responsibility of determining what can be done for patients and then doing it. Some patients are offered toileting assistance on a 2-hour schedule, and others are simply checked and changed. If patients are not offered toileting assistance, it is primarily because they cannot successfully use the toilet. The specific needs of patients are assessed, and an individualized incontinence management program is designed. See Appendix A for a sample of the form that can be used by a nursing home to communicate these points.

In summary, nursing homes must provide basic incontinence management. The problem cannot be ignored because of misunderstanding and lack of knowledge on the part of caring but misguided family members. The following chapter describes the two basic incontinence-management strategies that should be the primary responsibility of any good nursing service.

REFERENCE

American Health Care Association. (1987). *The long term care survey.* Washington, DC: Health Care Financing Administration. (Catalog No. 110334/12-87/5M1BAL)

Chapter 3

BASIC INCONTINENCE MANAGEMENT

What to learn from this chapter:

1. **What two incontinence management procedures form the basis of incontinence care.**
2. **What the different toileting program strategies are.**
3. **What the prompted-voiding toileting strategy is and why it should be used.**
4. **What the steps in prompted-voiding management are.**
5. **What the check–change management strategy is.**

All incontinent patients must be kept as dry as possible. This dryness goal can be accomplished with one of two basic nurse management procedures. One depends on frequent toileting assistance, whereas the other provides for frequent changing. All incontinent patients must receive one of these procedures as the minimum basis of care.

In some cases patients may also receive medical or behavioral treatment to supplement basic toileting or changing management. This supplementary treatment is most successful when substantial individual contact between caregivers and patients is possible. In home-care settings, other treatment options may prove useful in supplementing the two basic procedures. In nursing home situations, where there are many incontinent patients and relatively few caregivers, the two basic management procedures provide the primary focus of incontinence care. This chapter describes these two basic programs: toileting and changing.

TOILETING MANAGEMENT

The logic of toileting management programs suggests that if patients are taught to void frequently in toileting receptacles they will not be incontinent between toileting opportunities. This logic holds true only if patients can do two things: (a) start the voiding process if given access to a toilet and (b) hold urine during intervals between toiletings. Many patients have these abilities and will thus benefit from toileting management procedures. Three types of toileting management procedures can be identified: (1) timed voiding, (2) scheduled toileting, and (3) prompted voiding.

Timed voiding programs involve, first, identifying specific times a patient is likely to void. Efforts are then made to schedule toileting opportunities around these times. Presumably, time is saved because staff need to make contact with the patient only during those critical times when the patient is most in need.

Several major problems must be resolved if timed voiding programs are to work. First, the patient's schedule of voiding must be established, and it must be predictable. Unfortunately, predictable voiding schedules cannot be identified for many patients. It is therefore impossible to specify a critical time in which toileting assistance opportunities would be most successful.

The second problem arises even if individualized patient voiding schedules can be identified: it is difficult for staff to remember a variety of patient schedules. The nature of nurse's aides' work demands does not easily accommodate multiple, individualized patient-contact strategies.

Scheduled-toileting programs are simpler to manage than timed voiding programs. Scheduled programs involve contacting the patient on a fixed time schedule (usually 2 hours) and providing toileting assistance. There are no specific communication steps that are followed in simple scheduled-toileting protocols, and how the staff induces patients to toilet is left unspecified. In most cases, patients are toileted with minimal preparation or verbal interaction. Toileting becomes a habit or routine in which the patient plays a passive role.

Prompted voiding is also a scheduled-toileting program, but one with a communication protocol. Aides are trained to talk to patients in a specific and directed manner. These communication steps help reduce patient passivity and facilitate the toileting process. Efforts are made to encourage patients to take more responsibility and to request toileting assistance. Thus, prompted voiding is a scheduled-toileting program with a communication difference.

Prompted voiding takes little more time than simple scheduled toileting, but it involves a more mature and humane interaction with patients. At worst, aides will not verbally interact well with patients, and prompted voiding will be reduced to a simple scheduled toilet protocol. At best, verbal interaction will produce a more responsible, dry, and energetic patient.

PROMPTED VOIDING

Five steps comprise the prompted-voiding process: check, talk, prompt, praise, and correct. These steps are illustrated in Figure 3.1.

Check

The prompted-voiding process begins with a physical check of patients' linens. Before this check, patients should be called by name and told that their clothes are going to be checked for wetness or dryness. The checking process can prove deceptively difficult. Checking procedures in which patients are not physically repositioned often result in many missed wet checks.

It is impossible to detect wet checks consistently if staff attempt to feel wetness by simply running their hands under patients' clothes. This is particularly true for heavy patients or patients who are in a sitting position. Patients who are in a sitting position should be helped to stand up and their pads or diapers removed for inspection. Patients in a lying position should be gently rolled.

Checks will normally occur on a 2-hour schedule. The 2-hour repositioning required during the checks should not be stressful to patients. In fact, moving patients every 2 hours is considered good general nursing care.

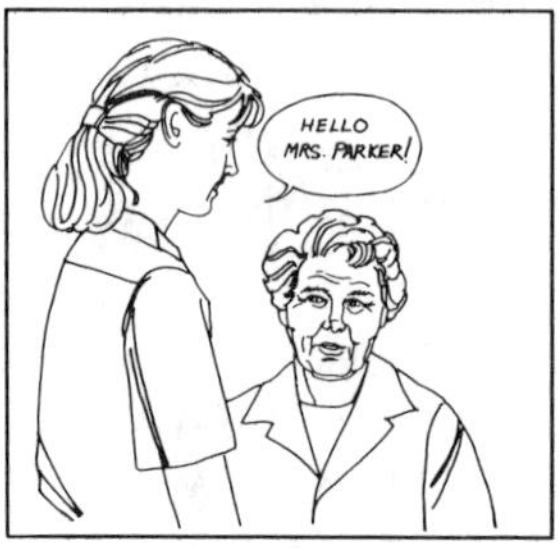

1. Always greet the resident by name. (Remember to always knock for resident privacy. Close the door and/or privacy curtain.)

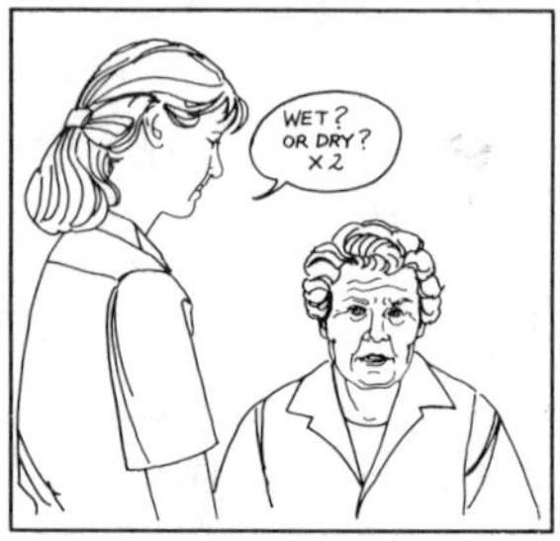

2. Ask the resident if he/she is wet or dry. Ask a second time if the resident doesn't respond.

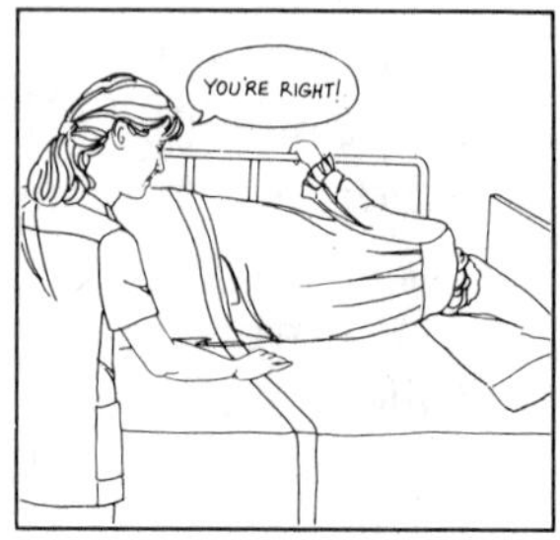

3. Turn or reposition the resident and check clothes, bedding, or body to determine if he/she is wet or dry. Tell the resident if he/she is correct.

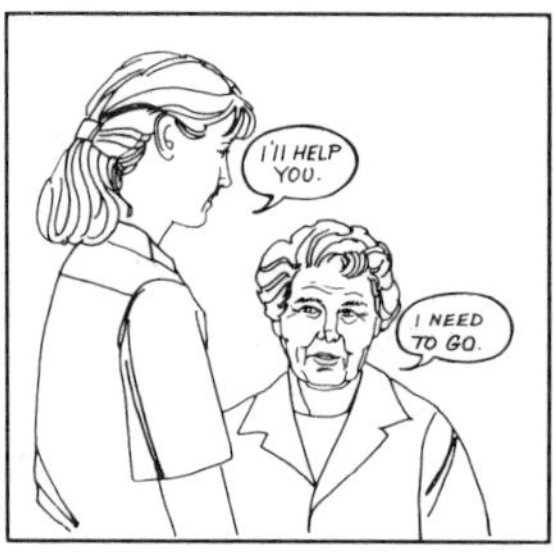

4. If the resident asks for help in toileting:
a. Praise the resident.
b. Assist him/her to toilet.

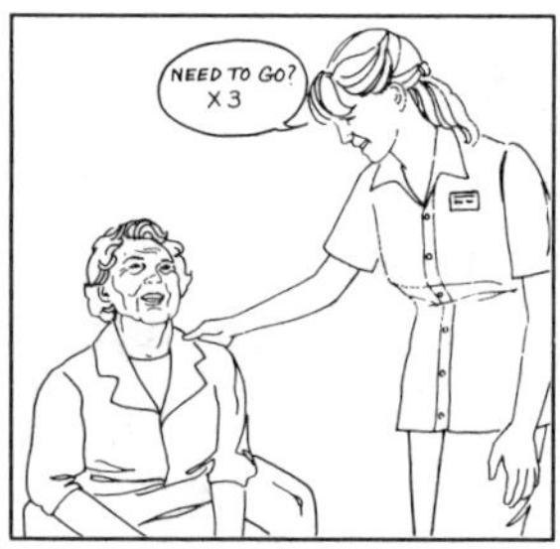

5. If the resident does not ask for help in toileting, YOU ask the resident if he/she wants to toilet.
a. Ask the resident again if he/she doesn't say yes the first time.
b. Ask the resident a third time if his/her response is other than yes or no.

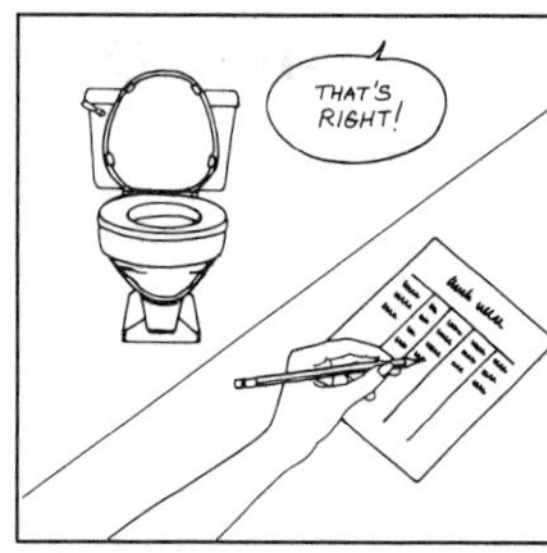

6. Assist resident to toilet only if he/she says yes to your offer.
a. Praise the resident for appropriate toileting.
b. Record outcome.

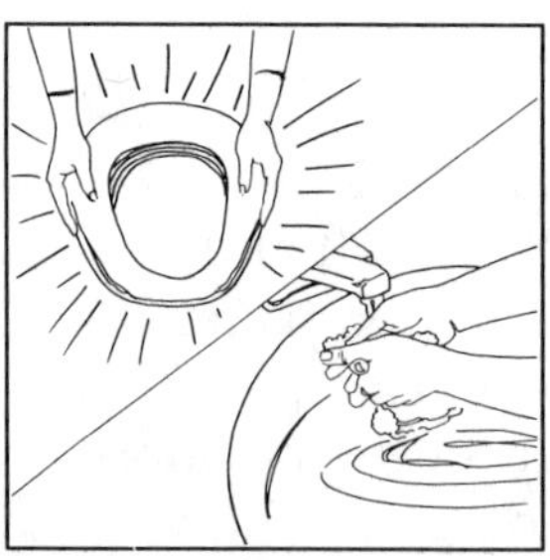

7. Empty and clean bedpan, urinal, or commode. Wash your hands. (Use your facility's infection control guidelines for handling urine and BM.)

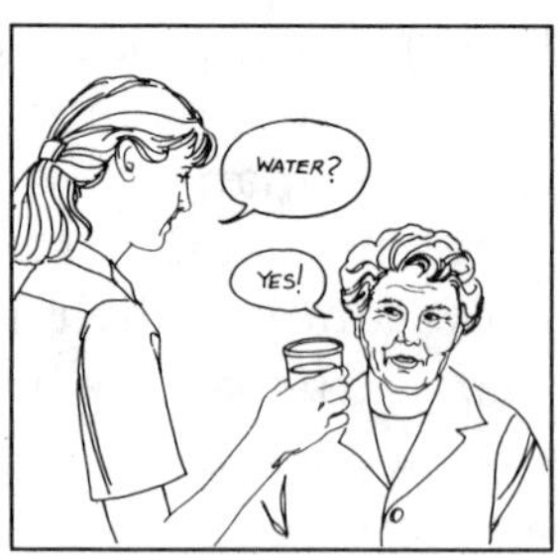

8. Ask the resident if he/she wants a drink of water, and give it if he/she says yes.

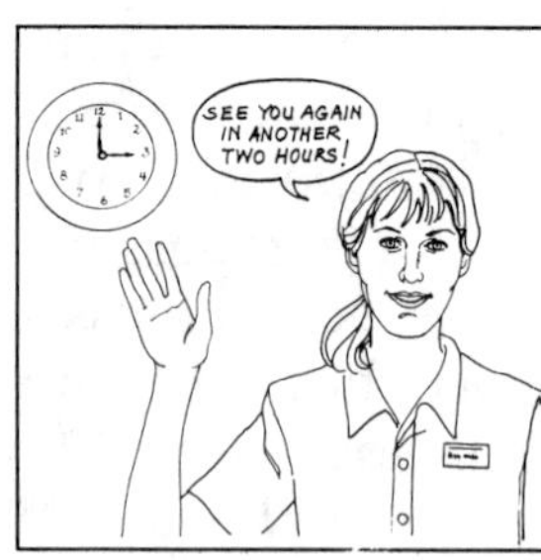

9. Tell the resident when he/she can expect you to be back.

FIGURE 3.1 Steps in the prompted-voiding protocol.

Talk

After determining whether the patient is wet or dry, the staff member should encourage the patient to talk about his or her continence status. Immediately after the check and before the patient is changed, the patient should be asked "Mrs. X, are you wet or dry?" If the patient does not answer the first time, the question should be repeated, up to three times. If the patient does answer the question, the staff person should give feedback about the accuracy of the patient's answer. For example, if patients are dry and say they are dry, they should be told something like "That's right, Mrs. X, you are dry. That's good." If patients are wet and say they are wet, then similar feedback concerning the accuracy of their answer should be given. For example, the staff member may say, "That's right, Mrs. X, you are wet." The purpose of this question and of the resulting interaction is to involve the patient in the incontinence care process.

Even patients with severe memory impairments should be able to answer questions about their current wet or dry status. Efforts to get patients to recognize whether they are wet or dry is a fundamental step to increase patients' awareness about their condition.

These wet/dry questions are also the most valid mental responsiveness screen that can be used to determine which patients are suitable for toileting programs and which are not. Some patients will be too mentally unresponsive to answer the question. They will respond with nonsensical answers or no answers at all. If a patient does not make a rational response after one day of asking this question every 2 hours, that patient should not be considered for a toileting program. Patients who make any attempt to answer the question (correctly or not) should not be screened from the toileting program even if they appear to have severe cognitive impairment. Attempts to answer the questions show that a patient has the minimal ability to understand verbal instructions. Such a basic ability is the fundamental skill needed to respond to the prompted-voiding program.

Prompt

After talking about the patient's continence status, the staff member asks if the patient will try to use the toileting receptacle. This step is called prompting and is repeated up to three times. Efforts should be made to be very persuasive during this process. If patients do not appear to understand the first prompt or if they appear uncertain as to what to do, aides should present the second, stronger prompt. For example, a typical prompting sequence may proceed as follows: First prompt: "Mrs. X, would you like to use the bathroom?" Mrs. X is uncertain and says, "Well, I don't know." Second prompt: "Mrs. X, maybe you had better try. I won't be back for two hours." Mrs. X responds with more uncertainty and shrugs her shoulders. Third prompt: "Mrs. X, please give it a try. What do you say?"

Patients are never toileted unless they answer yes to one of the prompts. Patients who cannot be persuaded to say yes to one of the prompts will generally be unresponsive even if they are automatically placed on the toilet. Alternatively, patients who can be brought to say yes are much more likely to use the toileting receptacle successfully. Most important, as the training program proceeds, patients will be more decisive in their response to the prompts. The prompt process will eventually take less time, and patients will take more responsibility for their toileting needs. Like the talking process, the purpose of the prompting process is to involve patients actively in the toileting program. The prompting process, like the questions concerning wetness or dryness, is designed to encourage patients to take more responsibility for their condition.

Praise

Once prompting is completed, patients are praised for either of two reasons: (a) they made an effort to use the toilet or (b) they were dry. Statements such as "Very good, Mrs. X, you tried to use the bathroom" should be made even if the patient tries to use the toilet but cannot void. If patients are dry and refuse the prompts, they should still be praised with a statement like "It is good that you stayed dry. I will be back in two more hours. Be sure to stay that way." This praise step helps ensure that patients understand that they are expected to stay dry and that they should try to toilet. This step is critical in reversing patients' lack of concern and passivity regarding their incontinence.

Correction

In a case where the patient is wet, there should be something said to support the expectation that the patient stay dry. For example, an appropriate corrective statement would be "You were wet, Mrs. X. I hope you will ask me before you have to go the next time." If the patient is wet but still tries to use the toilet by responding yes to a prompt, the staff member should place less emphasis on this corrective feedback. Instead, the patient should be praised for attempting to use the toilet.

CHANGING MANAGEMENT

Only about 35% to 50% of all incontinent patients can benefit from a toileting-assistance program. Toileting-responsive patients can and must be separated from unresponsive patients during a brief assessment period. Assessment procedures are described in Chapter 4.

The primary management procedure for patients not responsive to the toileting program must have as its goal keeping patients maximally dry. This basic management protocol is called the check–change protocol; patients are physically checked every 2 hours using the same procedures employed during prompted voiding. Physical repositioning of patients remains an important step in this checking process.

Patients should also be talked to during the check–change process. The talk, however, should be general and not related to the patient's incontinence condition. Questions concerning wetness or dryness are not appropriate because patients on a check–change protocol will not be able to control their voiding frequency; therefore, such questions may be frustrating. These patients, of course, are not prompted to toilet, and neither praise nor corrective feedback is given concerning their wetness or dryness. Steps in the check–change protocol are listed in Figure 3.2.

For most patients a change will be necessary approximately every 2 hours. This check–change schedule can be individualized for some people during the day and for many patients during the

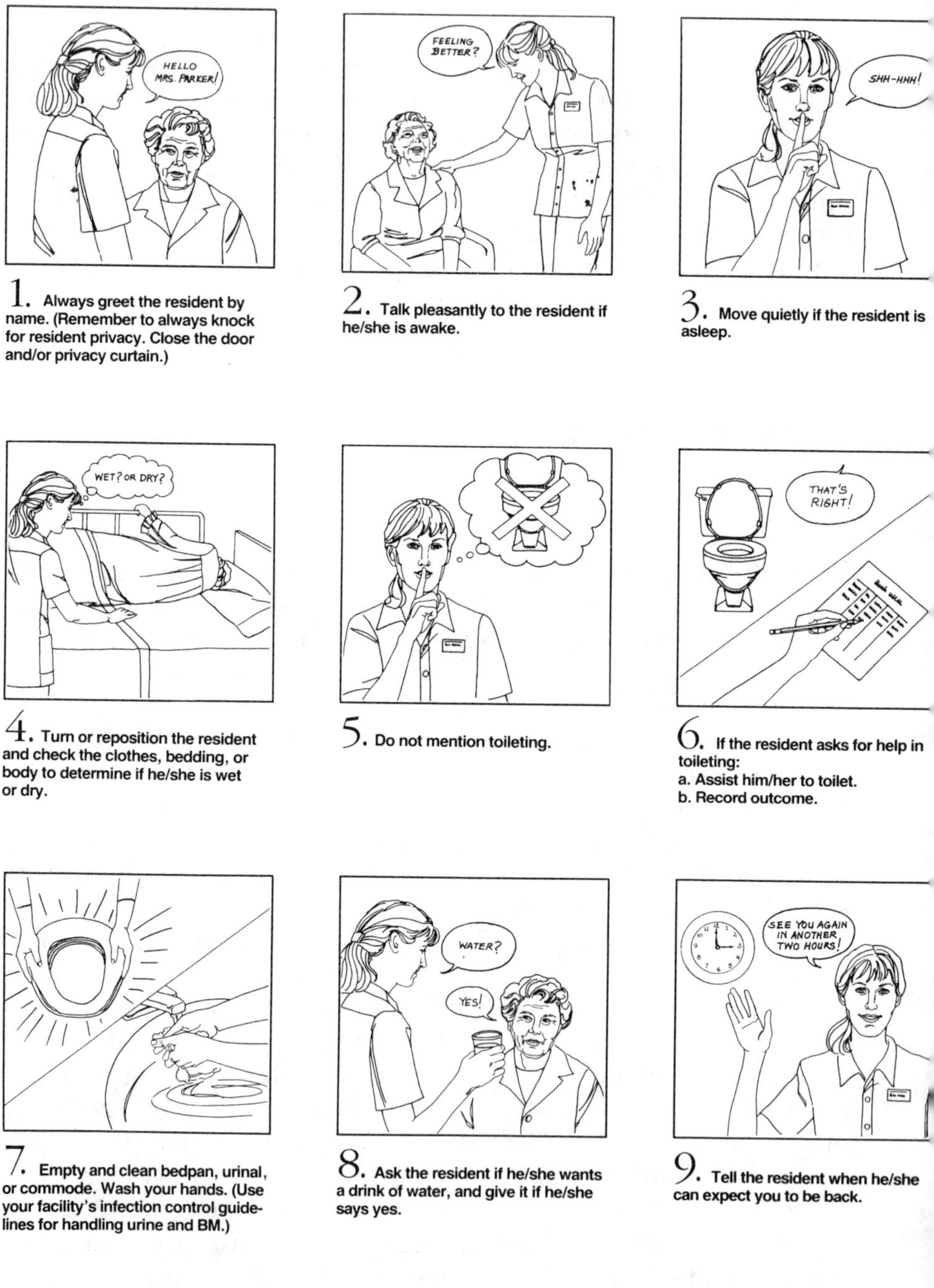

1. Always greet the resident by name. (Remember to always knock for resident privacy. Close the door and/or privacy curtain.)

2. Talk pleasantly to the resident if he/she is awake.

3. Move quietly if the resident is asleep.

4. Turn or reposition the resident and check the clothes, bedding, or body to determine if he/she is wet or dry.

5. Do not mention toileting.

6. If the resident asks for help in toileting:
a. Assist him/her to toilet.
b. Record outcome.

7. Empty and clean bedpan, urinal, or commode. Wash your hands. (Use your facility's infection control guidelines for handling urine and BM.)

8. Ask the resident if he/she wants a drink of water, and give it if he/she says yes.

9. Tell the resident when he/she can expect you to be back.

FIGURE 3.2 Steps in the check–change protocol.

night. Some patients will show frequent but small voids during the day. These patients will be wet often but not very wet. They are ideal for a padding system that is heavily absorbent (i.e., adult diapers). The use of such absorbent material to control small incontinence volumes will save time because patients will not need to be changed every 2 hours. These incontinent patients may be safely changed once or twice per shift.

Monitoring patients' incontinence volume over time permits staff to identify those who should be considered for an individualized changing program. How this monitoring can be done is discussed in Chapter 4, "Assessment."

During the night (11:00 P.M. to 7:00 A.M.), there should be a major effort to individualize the change schedule for some patients so as to minimally disrupt sleep. Individualization of nighttime incontinence-management schedules is extremely important. How and why such nighttime change schedules can be individualized is discussed specifically in Chapter 7.

Chapter **4**

ASSESSMENT

What to learn from this chapter:

1. **How to assess and select patients for either *toileting* or *changing* management.**
2. **How to summarize assessment information so as to justify the treatment decision.**
3. **How to measure appropriate toileting ability and why appropriate toileting is important.**
4. **How to screen patients with cognitive impairment.**
5. **How to identify patients who cannot hold urine for 2-hour intervals.**

A meaningful assessment of patients' responsiveness to a toileting program can be completed in one 12-hour day. A more complete assessment, permitting the design of more precise quality-control systems, requires 6 days. Since the assessment procedures are neither painful nor unusually time-consuming, the 6-day assessment period is recommended. Procedures utilized on each of the 6 assessment days are described separately. Thus, care providers who choose a 1-day assessment should implement only the first-day assessment procedures.

Procedures described in this chapter are designed for nursing homes and home settings where the elderly patient is frail or incapable of independent toileting. Assessment procedures for more mentally competent elderly patients, who also can toilet independently, are described in Chapter 8.

ASSESSMENT OBJECTIVES

The primary objective of the assessment period is to separate patients who can benefit from a toileting program from those who cannot. Patients who cannot benefit from scheduled toiletings must be placed on a well-managed changing program. A related objective is to develop information that can be used to control the quality of either incontinence program. Finally, a complete assessment system will provide data useful in developing individualized treatment programs to supplement the two primary management programs: toileting and changing.

Assessment data will answer the following major questions: What is the patient's normal voiding frequency? What is the patient's normal volume of voiding during continent and incontinent episodes? What is the patient's ability to answer simple questions related to incontinence? Will the patient attempt to use a toilet receptacle, and can the patient initiate voiding when given access to a receptacle? Can the patient store urine for at least 2 hours between checks?

Because of time and resource limitations it is important to collect the data most appropriate to a patient's future incontinence management. Thus, if patients will be managed with a check–change program, quality-control data relevant to managing that program must be emphasized during the assessment period. Alternatively, if patients are to be managed by a toileting program, the assessment period should emphasize that type of quality-control data.

A basic decision following each assessment day involves the question, will patients continue to be assessed for toileting management or changing management? Guidelines for making this decision are discussed after a description of the protocol for each assessment day.

PREPARATION FOR FIRST ASSESSMENT DAY

Two to three nurse's aides should be trained in the assessment protocols. The aides will implement simple assessment procedures, but it is vital that those procedures be implemented consistently. Aides selected for this training should have a history of accurate data recording. Aide training can best be accomplished if a professional nurse works with the aides during the first 3 assessment days. The professional nurse should be able to provide good training after reading this book.

One aide can successfully assess five to six patients if he or she is assigned full-time to the assessment task. If only one patient is to be assessed, aides can be assigned a normal patient-care load. The basic materials needed to begin each assessment day are listed in Appendix B along with all other forms needed to complete the assessment process.

ASSESSMENT DAY 1

All assessment days begin at 7:00 A.M. Patients are checked for wetness and placed in preweighed diapers or pads. Diapers are preferred because of their ability to contain urine. However, if patients object to diapering, a preweighed pad is acceptable.

The entire prompted-voiding procedure (see Chapter 3) is implemented with all patients at 7:00 A.M. All relevant information on the Day 1 Assessment Form is recorded. This form is illustrated in Figure 4.1.

It is important to note that the 7:00 A.M. information is not used to make decisions concerning patients' suitability for toileting management. If patients are wet at 7:00 A.M., it cannot be known when wetness occurred or if patients had an opportunity to toilet before the wetness. In short, nighttime incontinence differs from daytime incontinence and must be analyzed separately.

The first usable assessment data are collected at 9:00 A.M. Throughout the first assessment day, patients should be checked and prompted every 2 hours. Thus, checks will be completed at 9:00 A.M., 11:00 A.M., 1:00 P.M., 3:00 P.M., 5:00 P.M., and 7:00 P.M. Data are summarized after the 7:00 P.M. check.

The most important data used to make decisions about patients after this first assessment day are reflected by the responsiveness column on the Day 1 Assessment Form (Figure 4.1). This critical decision point is summarized at the bottom of Figure 4.1.

If patients attempted to answer even one question about their wetness or dryness, they should be assessed with the prompted-voiding procedure on the second day. It is not necessary that patients be accurate in response to the question "Are you wet or are you dry?" If patients make no attempt to answer the question,

Patient Name Smith
Nurse's Name Brown
Date ______

Checks	Wetness		Toileting		Responsiveness			Volume	
No. of checks made	Patient was (Circle one)		Did patient use the toilet? Yes: Urine or BM No: No attempt		Did patient answer question of wet or dry? (Circle One)			CC of void	
7:00 A.M.	**(wet)**	dry	yes	**(no)**	yes correct	**(yes incorrect)**	no answer	cont.	incont.
9:00 A.M.	**(wet)**	dry	**(yes)**	no	yes correct	**(yes incorrect)**	no answer	cont. 125	incont. 50
11:00 A.M.	wet	**(dry)**	yes	**(no)**	**(yes correct)**	yes incorrect	no answer	cont.	incont.
1:00 P.M.	wet	**(dry)**	yes	**(no)**	yes correct	**(yes incorrect)**	no answer	cont.	incont.
3:00 P.M.	**(wet)**	dry	**(yes)**	no	yes correct	**(yes incorrect)**	no answer	cont. 10	incont. 20
5:00 P.M.	wet	**(dry)**	yes	**(no)**	**(yes correct)**	yes incorrect	no answer	cont.	incont.
7:00 P.M.	**(wet)**	dry	yes	**(no)**	yes correct	**(yes incorrect)**	no answer	cont.	incont. 20

Summary	Total number of wets	Total number of toilets	Total # correct	Total # incorrect	Total # no answer	Total cont. cc	Total incont. cc
9:00 A.M. to 7:00 P.M.	3	2	2	4	0	135	90

$$\frac{2}{3 + 2} = 40\ \%\ \text{Appropriate toileting}$$

Decision Point:

If there are any "Yes" responses in either Toileting or Responsiveness columns, continue patient on prompted voiding for the second day. If there are no "Yes" responses, put patient on check-change protocol. Calculate % Appropriate Toilets by dividing Total # of Toilets by Total # of wets + Total # of Toilets.

FIGURE 4.1 Day 1 Assessment Form.

they should be assessed with the check–change protocol on the second and all following assessment days. Patient response does not have to be verbal. If patients are nonverbal, some acknowledgment of their condition, such as nodding the head or blinking, could replace verbal response.

Patients who attempt no response to the questions are too disoriented or mentally impaired to respond to a scheduled-toileting or prompted-voiding program. The criteria for continuation in the prompted-voiding assessment becomes more rigid after each assessment day. During days 2 through 6, patients are asked to show some evidence of appropriate toileting ability to continue in prompted voiding.

A different assessment sheet is used to record information on each assessment day. The technician has only to answer each question on the sheet and summarize the data. The volume of continent voids is measured with a toileting insert, and incontinent volumes are measured by the difference in pre- and post-pad weights.

The numbers in the Day 1 Assessment Form (Figure 4.1) illustrate hypothetical data for Mrs. Smith. These numbers are discussed in the case study at the end of this chapter. In the example provided, the patient was wet at 7:00 A.M., 9:00 A.M., 3:00 P.M., and 7:00 P.M. The 7:00 A.M. point did not count and therefore was not summarized in the "Wet" column at the end of the day. There were appropriate toiletings at 9:00 A.M. and 3:00 P.M. Most important, the patient attempted to answer all questions concerning her wetness or dryness condition and was correct on two occasions. The decision was thus made to include the patient on prompted-voiding assessment for the second assessment day.

If the nursing home chooses not to assess further, the patient's appropriate toileting percentage should be calculated. The appropriate toileting percentage is an important statistic that measures the number of times patients use a toilet compared to total number of voids. Thus, totally continent patients exhibit a 100% appropriate toileting percentage. Patients who use a toilet four times and wet their clothes four times attain a 50% appropriate toileting rate: (4 appropriate toileting/4 appropriate toileting + 4 incontinent episodes).

If patients' appropriate toileting rates are above 75%, they should be managed with the prompted-voiding protocol. Patients whose appropriate toileting rate is below 75% should be managed with the check–change protocol. In the case illustrated in Figure 4.1 the patient's appropriate toileting percentage was 40%. If no further assessment is conducted, this patient should be managed with a check–change protocol.

ASSESSMENT DAY 2

The major difference between Assessment Day 1 and Day 2 is that during Day 2 some patients are on the check–change protocol (chapter 3) and some patients continue on the prompted-voiding protocol. The major difference with the check–change protocol is that subjects are not prompted to toilet and they are not asked, "Are you wet or dry?" Thus, the responsiveness column on the basic assessment data sheet is not used for patients on the check–change protocol. Appropriate toileting is recorded for check–change patients only if patients request assistance without being prompted. Once again, checks are conducted every 2 hours, starting at 7:00 A.M., and all information is summarized at the end of the day.

A second patient decision is made at the end of the second assessment day. This decision is based on two criteria: (1) patients should show a continuing effort to answer questions about their wetness or dryness (a score of at least one yes in the response column), and (2) there should be at least one appropriate toileting recorded in the toileting column. Successful appropriate toileting means that patients not only attempt to use a toilet receptacle but use the receptacle successfully.

All patients who show some score other than zero in those two areas should continue in the prompted-voiding assessment period for Days 3 and 4. Other patients are placed on the check–change protocol. In the case of the patient illustrated in the Day 2 Assessment Form, the decision is made to continue prompted voiding for the next 2 days (see Figure 4.2). This patient had three appropriate toiletings and attempted to answer the wet/dry question six times.

Patient Name Smith
Nurse's Name Brown
Date ______

Checks	Wetness		Toileting		Responsiveness			Volume	
No. of checks made	Patient was (Circle one)		Did patient use the toilet? Yes: Urine or BM No: No attempt		Did patient answer question of wet or dry? (Circle One)			CC of void	
7:00 A.M.	wet	dry	yes	no	yes correct	yes incorrect	no answer	cont.	incont.
9:00 A.M.	wet	dry	yes	no	yes correct	yes incorrect	no answer	cont. 125	incont.
11:00 A.M.	wet	dry	yes	no	yes correct	yes incorrect	no answer	cont.	incont.
1:00 P.M.	wet	dry	yes	no	yes correct	yes incorrect	no answer	cont. 25	incont.
3:00 P.M.	wet	dry	yes	no	yes correct	yes incorrect	no answer	cont.	incont. 15
5:00 P.M.	wet	dry	yes	no	yes correct	yes incorrect	no answer	cont.	incont.
7:00 P.M.	wet	dry	yes	no	yes correct	yes incorrect	no answer	cont. 230	incont. 25

Summary	Total number of wets	Total number of toilets	Total # correct	Total # incorrect	Total # no answer	Total cont. cc	Total incont. cc
9:00 A.M. to 7:00 P.M.	2	3	5	1	0	380	40

$$\frac{3}{2 + 3} = \underline{60}\ \%\ \text{Appropriate toileting}$$

Decision Point:

There must be a "Yes" response in both Toileting or Responsiveness columns. If so, continue patient on prompted voiding for the third day. If there is not a "Yes" response in both columns put patient on check-change protocol.

FIGURE 4.2 Day 2 Assessment Form.

ASSESSMENT DAYS 3 AND 4

No further decisions concerning patients are made until after Assessment Day 4. Thus, patients who continue prompted voiding after Day 2 should receive the prompted voiding protocol for both Day 3 and Day 4. Those patients on the check–change protocol should receive that protocol on both Day 3 and Day 4. The information for these 2 days is then summarized, and a decision is made concerning assessment Days 5 and 6.

Once again, criteria for continuing patients on the prompted-voiding protocol is made more precise. Patients should now show a minimum appropriate toileting percentage of 50% to continue prompted-voiding assessment. This means that half of all of their voids are successfully made into a toileting receptacle. Patients with rates below 50% are better candidates for the check–change protocol, and their incontinence should be evaluated with that protocol for Days 5 and 6.

The assessment forms for Days 3 and 4 (Figures 4.3 and 4.4) illustrate an example of a patient who met the criteria for continuing prompted voiding. This patient's appropriate toilet percentage was 67%.

ASSESSMENT DAYS 5 AND 6

Assessment procedures remain the same for patients during Days 5 and 6. One final decision remains after Day 6 for patients who continue on prompted voiding for the full 6-day period: Should patients' future treatment involve toileting management, or would they be better managed with a changing program? All patients who have finished the 6 days of prompted voiding show at least some toileting responsiveness. The question remains: Has enough toileting responsiveness been shown to justify ongoing toileting management?

One part of this decision is easy. All patients who show appropriate toileting rates above 75% during the last 2 days, or during the whole period, should continue in a prompted-voiding pro-

Patient Name Smith
Nurse's Name Brown
Date ______

Checks	Wetness		Toileting		Responsiveness			Volume	
No. of checks made	Patient was (Circle one)		Did patient use the toilet? Yes: Urine or BM No: No attempt		Did patient answer question of wet or dry? (Circle One)			CC of void	
7:00 A.M.	**wet**	dry	yes	**no**	**yes correct**	yes incorrect	no answer	cont.	incont.
9:00 A.M.	**wet**	dry	**yes**	no	**yes correct**	yes incorrect	no answer	cont. 50	incont. 30
11:00 A.M.	wet	**dry**	**yes**	no	**yes correct**	yes incorrect	no answer	cont. 75	incont.
1:00 P.M.	wet	**dry**	yes	**no**	**yes correct**	yes incorrect	no answer	cont.	incont.
3:00 P.M.	**wet**	dry	**yes**	no	**yes correct**	yes incorrect	no answer	cont. 80	incont. 35
5:00 P.M.	wet	**dry**	yes	**no**	**yes correct**	yes incorrect	no answer	cont.	incont.
7:00 P.M.	wet	**dry**	**yes**	no	**yes correct**	yes incorrect	no answer	cont. 120	incont.

Summary	Total number of wets	Total number of toilets	Total # correct	Total # incorrect	Total # no answer	Total cont. cc	Total incont. cc
9:00 A.M. to 7:00 P.M.	2	4	6	0	___	325	65

$$\frac{4}{2 + 4} = 67\ \%\ \text{Appropriate toileting}$$

Decision Point:
No decisions: continue prompted voiding patients on prompted void protocol. Continue check-change patients on check-change protocol.

FIGURE 4.3 Day 3 Assessment Form.

Patient Name Smith

Nurse's Name Brown

Date ______

Checks	Wetness		Toileting		Responsiveness			Volume	
No. of checks made	Patient was (Circle one)		Did patient use the toilet? Yes: Urine or BM No: No attempt		Did patient answer question of wet or dry? (Circle One)			CC of void	
7:00 A.M.	wet	**dry**	yes	**no**	**yes correct**	yes incorrect	no answer	cont.	incont.
9:00 A.M.	wet	**dry**	**yes**	no	**yes correct**	yes incorrect	no answer	cont. 150	incont.
11:00 A.M.	wet	**dry**	yes	**no**	**yes correct**	yes incorrect	no answer	cont.	incont.
1:00 P.M.	**wet**	dry	**yes**	no	**yes correct**	yes incorrect	no answer	cont. 75	incont. 40
3:00 P.M.	wet	**dry**	**yes**	no	**yes correct**	yes incorrect	no answer	cont. 90	incont.
5:00 P.M.	wet	**dry**	**yes**	no	**yes correct**	yes incorrect	no answer	cont. 85	incont.
7:00 P.M.	**wet**	dry	yes	**no**	**yes correct**	yes incorrect	no answer	cont.	incont. 50

Summary	Total number of wets	Total number of toilets	Total # correct	Total # incorrect	Total # no answer	Total cont. cc	Total incont. cc
9:00 A.M. to 7:00 P.M.	2	4	6	0	0	250	90

$$\frac{4}{2 + 4} = 67\ \%\ \text{Appropriate toileting}$$

Decision Point:

Patient must show an appropriate toilet percentage of 50% to continue in Prompted Voiding. Below 50% toileting should go to check-change protocol.

FIGURE 4.4 Day 4 Assessment Form.

Patient Name Smith

Nurse's Name Brown

Date ____________

Checks	Wetness		Toileting		Responsiveness			Volume	
No. of checks made	Patient was (Circle one)		Did patient use the toilet? Yes: Urine or BM No: No attempt		Did patient answer question of wet or dry? (Circle One)			CC of void	
7:00 A.M.	wet	**dry**	yes	**no**	**yes correct**	yes incorrect	no answer	cont.	incont.
9:00 A.M.	**wet**	dry	**yes**	no	**yes correct**	yes incorrect	no answer	cont. 125	incont. 80
11:00 A.M.	wet	**dry**	**yes**	no	**yes correct**	yes incorrect	no answer	cont. 75	incont.
1:00 P.M.	wet	**dry**	yes	**no**	**yes correct**	yes incorrect	no answer	cont.	incont.
3:00 P.M.	wet	**dry**	**yes**	no	**yes correct**	yes incorrect	no answer	cont. 90	incont.
5:00 P.M.	wet	**dry**	**yes**	no	**yes correct**	yes incorrect	no answer	cont. 120	incont.
7:00 P.M.	wet	**dry**	**yes**	no	**yes correct**	yes incorrect	no answer	cont. 150	incont.

Summary	Total number of wets	Total number of toilets	Total # correct	Total # incorrect	Total # no answer	Total cont. cc	Total incont. cc
9:00 A.M. to 7:00 P.M.	1	5	6	0	0	560	80

5 / (1 + 5) = 83 % Appropriate toileting

Decision Point:

No decision: continue prompted voiding patients in prompted voiding and check-change patient in check-change protocol.

FIGURE 4.5 Day 5 Assessment Form.

gram. Decisions about patients in the intermediate range of appropriate toileting (50% to 75%) are more difficult and depend on factors other than toileting ability.

In the patient data for Days 5 and 6 (Figures 4.5 and 4.6) it is clear that this patient's appropriate toileting ability is sufficient to allow for prompted-voiding management. The patient's appropriate toileting percentage during the last 2 days of prompted voiding was 83% on both days.

FINAL DATA SUMMARY

The flow chart in Figure 4.7 summarizes the assessment days described above. How and why patients are separated into toileting or check–change protocols during the 6 assessment days is illustrated clearly. Major decisions about patients are made after Day 1, Day 2, Day 4, and Day 6.

All assessment data should be summarized on the final assessment summary sheet and treatment decision form (Figure 4.8). This form provides documentation that a valid patient-incontinence assessment was performed. In addition, the form describes the data base justifying the treatment decision. It also provides a description of the three areas that are critical for patients' success in a toileting program: toileting ability, bladder storage ability, and responsiveness. Data from the patient are assessed with both the check–change and prompted-voiding protocols and should be summarized on the form.

The 6 days of assessment data shown in Figures 4.1–4.6 are summarized in Figure 4.8. The example patient had 12 wets and 23 successful toileting during the 6 assessment days (this summary is represented in columns 1 and 2). The numbers are taken from the first two summary columns on each day's data sheet and are added together for a total of 35 voids (column 3). The patient's final appropriate toileting score is then calculated by dividing column 2 (number of appropriate toilets) by column 3 (total number of voids). In this case, 23 divided by 35 equals a 66% appropriate toileting rate.

To estimate storage ability, the number of wets (column 1) is

Patient Name Smith
Nurse's Name Brown
Date ______

Checks	Wetness		Toileting		Responsiveness			Volume	
No. of checks made	Patient was (Circle one)		Did patient use the toilet? Yes: Urine or BM No: No attempt		Did patient answer question of wet or dry? (Circle One)			CC of void	
7:00 A.M.	wet	dry	yes	no	yes correct	yes incorrect	no answer	cont.	incont.
9:00 A.M.	wet	dry	yes	no	yes correct	yes incorrect	no answer	cont. 190	incont.
11:00 A.M.	wet	dry	yes	no	yes correct	yes incorrect	no answer	cont.	incont. 25
1:00 P.M.	wet	dry	yes	no	yes correct	yes incorrect	no answer	cont. 75	incont.
3:00 P.M.	wet	dry	yes	no	yes correct	yes incorrect	no answer	cont. 90	incont.
5:00 P.M.	wet	dry	yes	no	yes correct	yes incorrect	no answer	cont. 120	incont.
7:00 P.M.	wet	dry	yes	no	yes correct	yes incorrect	no answer	cont. 95	incont.

Summary	Total number of wets	Total number of toilets	Total # correct	Total # incorrect	Total # no answer	Total cont. cc	Total incont. cc
9:00 A.M. to 7:00 P.M.	1	5	6	0	0	570	25

$$\frac{5}{1 + 5} = 83 \text{ \% Appropriate toileting}$$

Decision Point:
Summarize all data on final assessment summary sheet.

FIGURE 4.6 Day 6 Assessment Form.

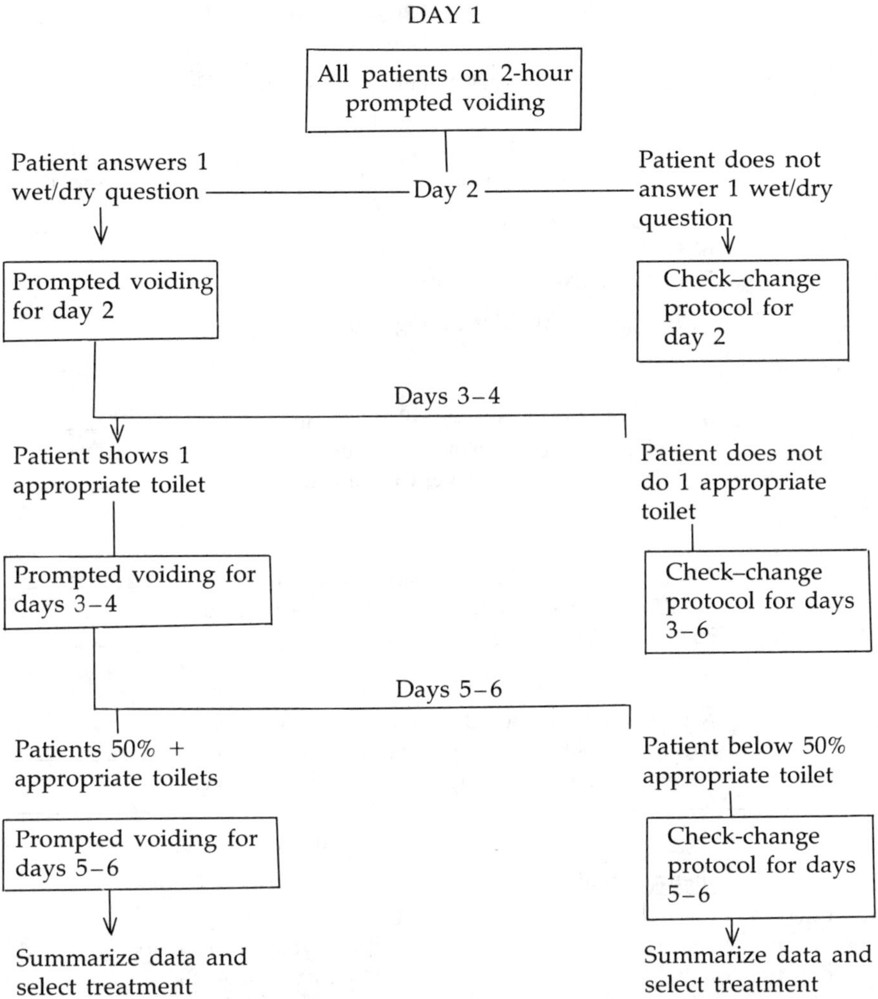

FIGURE 4.7 Flow chart of assessment days.

divided by the 6 assessment days. The 12 wets divided by 6 days equals 2 wets per day. The patient's average volume of incontinence episodes is calculated by summarizing the 6 days of incontinence volumes from the last column of each assessment sheet. A look at Figures 4.1–4.6 reveals that this patient had total daily incontinence volumes of 90 cc, 40 cc, 65 cc, 90 cc, 80 cc, and 25 cc, totaling 390 cc. This 390 cc total is divided by the total

Patient's Name ____________
Date ____________

Final Assessment Summary Sheet and Treatment Decision

Toileting Ability

Appropriate Toileting %	Check Appr. Box
0%–65% Poor ability to toilet	
66%–75% Average ability to toilet	X
75%–100% Excellent ability to toilet	

Bladder Storage Ability

Frequency of wets per day:

0–1 Good ability to prevent incontinence	
1–2 Marginal ability to prevent incontinence	X
2+ Poor ability to prevent incontinence	

Volume of wets per day:

0–30 cc Good ability to control urine loss	X
30–75 cc Marginal ability to control urine loss	
75+ cc Poor ability to control urine loss	

Mental Responsiveness

No question answered—poor responsiveness	
Answered 50% correctly—marginal responsiveness	
Answered 75% correctly—excellent responsiveness	X

6-Day Assessment Summary

Toileting ability

Column
1 total no. wets 12
2 total no. toilets 23
3 total no. voids (columns 1 + 2) 35
4 % appr. toilet $\frac{\text{(column 2)}}{\text{(column 3)}}$ $\frac{23}{35} = .66$

Storage ability

5 No. expected wets per day $\frac{\text{(total wets)}}{6} =$ $\frac{12}{6} = 2$

6 Avg. vol. inc. episodes $\frac{\text{(add all inc. vols)}}{\text{(column 1)}} =$ $\frac{390}{12} = 32.5$

7 Lowest inc. vol 15
Largest Inc. vol 80

Responsiveness

Column
8 no. yes correct responses 31
9% correct $\frac{\text{(col. 8)}}{\text{no. days in prompted voiding} \times 6} =$ $\frac{31}{36} = 86$

FIGURE 4.8 Final assessment summary.

number of wets (column 1): 390 cc divided by 12 wets equals an average incontinence volume of 32.5 cc.

The patient's largest incontinence volume is also listed in column 8. These numbers are gathered by simply looking at each incontinence volume measured during each assessment day. In this case, the lowest incontinence volume was 15 cc on Day 2, and the highest was 80 cc on Day 5. These numbers prove useful in designing a quality-control system for patients placed in a changing program.

Finally, patients' mental responsiveness is evaluated by summarizing the total number of times patients answer the "wet or dry" question accurately (column 8), gathered from the "yes, correct" responsiveness column summary on each data assessment form. That number is divided by the total number of times the question was asked. The question is asked six times each day the patient is on a prompted-voiding protocol. Thus, if a patient was on the prompted-voiding for 6 days, the number of yes responses is divided by 36. The sample patient gave 31 correct responses. The question was asked 36 times, so the patient was correct 86% (31/36) of the time. The following case study provides a more complete description of the assessment process and the final treatment decision that is made based on the assessment data.

CASE STUDY—SMITH

Mrs. Smith is an 83-year-old patient recently admitted to a nursing facility from home. Her family and physician admitted her because of progressive deterioration in her ability to care for herself. She was unsteady and had fallen several times within the last 2 months. She could ambulate only with assistance because she could not lift herself from a chair to a standing position. She required the aid of a walker to actually ambulate.

Her memory was also poor. She could not remember the day of the week and could not recall the names of people she had just met. She had reached the point at which she required total supervision, and she had been incontinent for more than 6 months. At first the problem occurred only at night, but it worsened progressively during the day. Mrs. Smith attempted to control the problem by wearing adult diapers. She had not attempted to void in a toilet for over 3 months at the time of her admission.

Five days after Mrs. Smith's admission, the first incontinent assessment day was begun. Mrs. Smith was checked at 7:00 A.M., and her diaper was changed. Mrs. Smith was also asked if she was wet or dry. She did not understand the question at first and as a result did not respond. She was asked a second time and was confused as to what her answer should be so she said, "No, I'm not wet." She actually was wet, so Mrs. Smith scored incorrect in her answer to this question.

Next Mrs. Smith was asked if she would try to use the toilet. This surprised her because no one had asked her that question in over 3 months. She said yes and was taken to the bathroom. When she was placed on the commode, she could not initiate voiding. She had recently been incontinent and had little urine left in her bladder. Despite this dry run, the staff person praised her effort, placed her in a chair, and offered her a drink. Mrs. Smith's data were recorded in the 7:00 A.M. block, and she was told that the staff person would return in 2 hours.

During the 9:00 A.M. check the entire procedure was repeated. Mrs. Smith responded more quickly to the question "Are you wet or dry?" and this time said she was not wet. Once again, however, she was wrong. Prompted to try to use the bedpan, she responded with a yes and voided successfully. The urine was measured with a toileting insert; Mrs. Smith had a 125-cc void. Her wet diaper was weighed and found to contain 50 cc of urine. She was changed, praised for toileting, given a drink, and told that the staff person would return in 2 hours.

During the remainder of the day, Mrs. Smith was wet two more times (3:00 P.M. and 7:00 P.M.), but she did successfully void one more time at the 3:00 P.M. check. She attempted to answer all of the "Are you wet or dry" questions even though she was seldom correct. She did answer the question correctly at 11:00 A.M. and 5:00 P.M. Mrs. Smith's data were summarized at the end of the assessment day.

Mrs. Smith clearly showed potential. She exhibited enough responsiveness to try to answer the simple question, "Are you wet or dry?" which showed she had the mental capacity to recognize that she was being asked a question. More important, she showed an ability to initiate voiding twice during the first assessment day. Thus, Mrs. Smith met the criteria for continuing on prompted-voiding assessment for the second day.

Mrs. Smith's response for the second assessment day is illustrated by the data on the Day 2 Assessment Form (see Figure 4.2). She continued to show some improvement in her ability to answer the question "Are you wet or dry?" In fact, she answered correctly five of the six times she was asked. She was wet two times, but she continued to exhibit appropriate toileting ability. She appropriately toileted three times. The size of her incontinent voids were relatively small (15 cc at 3:00 P.M., 25 cc at 7:00 P.M.). By contrast, the size of her continent voids were larger (125 cc, 25 cc, and 230 cc). Her appropriate percentage was 60%. Mrs. Smith clearly showed the potential to continue on prompted voiding for the third and fourth assessment days.

During Days 3 and 4 she once again revealed some ability to answer questions and some ability to initiate voiding. She accurately answered the "Are you wet or dry?" question 100% of the time, and she had an appropriate toileting rate of 67%. Unfortunately, she continued to be wet about two times per 12-hour period. The voids continued to be small (30 cc and 35 cc on Day 3 and 40 cc and 50 cc on Day 4). Mrs. Smith met the criteria to continue on the prompted-voiding protocol for the remaining 2 days of the assessment period.

On the final 2 days, Mrs. Smith continued to show appropriate toileting ability. She was wet once on Day 5 and once on Day 6. Her appropriate toileting percentage was 83% on those 2 days. Mrs. Smith's data are summarized in the final data summary form shown in Figure 4.8.

Mrs. Smith should be managed with the toileting program because of average toileting ability and excellent responsiveness. Her overall appropriate toileting percentage was 66%, but her average in the last 2 days of the prompted-voiding assessment was 83%.

Her bladder storage ability is rated as only marginal because of the two wet episodes per day. Patients with better storage ability would be wet less than once per day. However, even this marginal rating must not be overemphasized. The patient's average volume of voiding was 32.5 cc. This is a low figure, but it suggests that the patient does have adequate storage ability to justify toileting program management. The patient was usually responsive. She answered 89% of the questions accurately.

SELECTING TOILETING OR CHANGING MANAGEMENT FOR PATIENTS

The most important statistic to consider when selecting the correct management program for a patient is appropriate toileting ability. If a patient has an appropriate toileting rate of 75% or more for the whole assessment period or the last 2 days, he or she should be managed with prompted voiding. Managers must look at factors other than appropriate toileting rates to decide on the management strategy for patients with appropriate toileting rates between 50% and 74%.

Two major problems arise if patients with appropriate toileting between 50% and 75% are placed on a toileting program. First, these patients will continue to be wet two or more times per 12-hour period. This continuing high wetness rate presents problems when managers attempt to control the quality of the toileting program. Second, these patients require both frequent toileting and changing assistance. Thus, they consume more staff time than patients with high appropriate toileting and low wet rates.

Despite the high wetness problems that characterize this 50%–75% appropriate toileting group, some patients will show important changes that a nurse manager must consider. For example, many patients will show a major reduction in the volume of their incontinence episodes. Thus, even though they are frequently wet, they are not extremely wet. The general rule follows that if patients' average wetness volumes per incontinence episode are 30 cc or lower, they will probably benefit from a toileting program. These patients will be much wetter if they are managed on a check–change protocol.

In addition, some patients in this subgroup will be easy and efficient to toilet. They will be easy because they are cooperative and enjoy the attention and interaction that surrounds the prompted-voiding protocol. They are efficient to work with because they successfully toilet most of the time that they request assistance. A good rule to follow is that if patients have a 50%–75% appropriate toileting rate and answer 75% of the wet/dry questions correctly, they are efficient to work with on the toileting program.

In general, the nurse manager must make a clinical decision concerning these patients. Staff resources, the success of the nursing home in maintaining other patients on a toileting program, and patient factors described in this section must all be considered. The decision will be easier to make after the nurse manager has some experience with the assessment program and with the ability of staff to maintain patients on a consistent schedule.

If the program is just getting started, it is probably a good idea to include only patients who show high responsiveness (75% and higher appropriate toileting rates). Marginal patients can be reevaluated for toileting management after it is clear that the nursing service is managed to the point that a consistent toileting schedule is maintained.

Alternatively, marginal patients may constitute a group in critical need of a medical consultant. These patients clearly demonstrate that they understand the voiding prompt and are motivated to toilet. Their 50%–75% toileting rate documents their abilities. Unfortunately, either bladder storage or bladder emptying problems prevent these promising patients from benefiting from simple toileting management. These patients may be ideal candidates for supplemental medical treatment.

Chapter 5

PROGRAM IMPLEMENTATION

What to learn from this chapter:

1. **How to document patient response to the incontinence program.**
2. **How to increase the accuracy of information recorded by aides.**
3. **How to train aides when the program starts.**
4. **How to identify and correct program start-up problems.**
5. **How to add new patients to the program.**
6. **When and how to reduce supervision.**

The first 3 days that a facility uses a program are critical. Aides must be taught new work habits in regard to both record keeping and patient care. Strong leadership is required during this period to prevent the problems often associated with nursing home rehabilitation programs.

Inaccurate or even false data recording by aides is one such problem that must be overcome. Unfortunately, many aides have learned that simply recording that patient care activities occurred is as good as actually performing the tasks. Good training solves only some of these difficulties because a large part of the problem is poor motivation. Aides may know what to do but fail to do it because it takes more time. This chapter describes how the incontinence program should be introduced and initially managed.

DOCUMENTATION PROCEDURES

Patients' response to a toileting program must be documented in order for facilities to meet federal standards for patient care. In addition to fulfilling these regulations a good documentation system serves an important management function. It keeps aides' attention on patient-care tasks. The "active" incontinence recording system described in this book is designed to achieve both patient documentation and management objectives. The system is called active because it requires more overt behavior than do traditional documentation systems. It requires more of each aide and floor supervisor than simply filling out a form.

The toileting chart or paper that is used to document patient incontinence progress is less important than the system within which the chart is used. An example of a clear and efficient toileting chart is illustrated in Figure 5.1, but caregivers can make their own chart as long as it contains the same type of information.

Hours are listed vertically in the chart, and symbols describing the patient's incontinence status are shown for each hour. The caregiver has only to put a (X) across the appropriate symbol. The chart should be used every 2 hours. If a patient is wet, a (X) is placed across either the small drop, symbolizing a small wet, or a large drop, indicating a large wet. If the patient is dry, a (X) is placed across the cactus. If the patient toilets successfully, a (X) should be placed on the symbol of the toilet. If volumes are being measured, an entry about the volume of the void can be made. The volume column is optional. The right-hand column, also optional, indicates whether or not the patient drank fluids.

Particularly important is the space left for a supervisor check. During the beginning stage of the program, the floor nurse should make one check on the patient per day. This check is made during times when nurses are normally in contact with patients (for example, during medicine-passing rounds). Floor supervisors should write the time of the check and note whether they found patients wet or dry. This can be signified by simply writing "w" or "d."

Finally, the floor nurse should check to see if aides are marking charts at the required 2-hour intervals. If there is a 3-hour block without an aide notation of patients' conditions, the supervisor should draw a bracket around the 3-hour block and call this omission to the aide's attention.

The quality assurance nurse will also make daily checks on patients during the first program week and should mark the

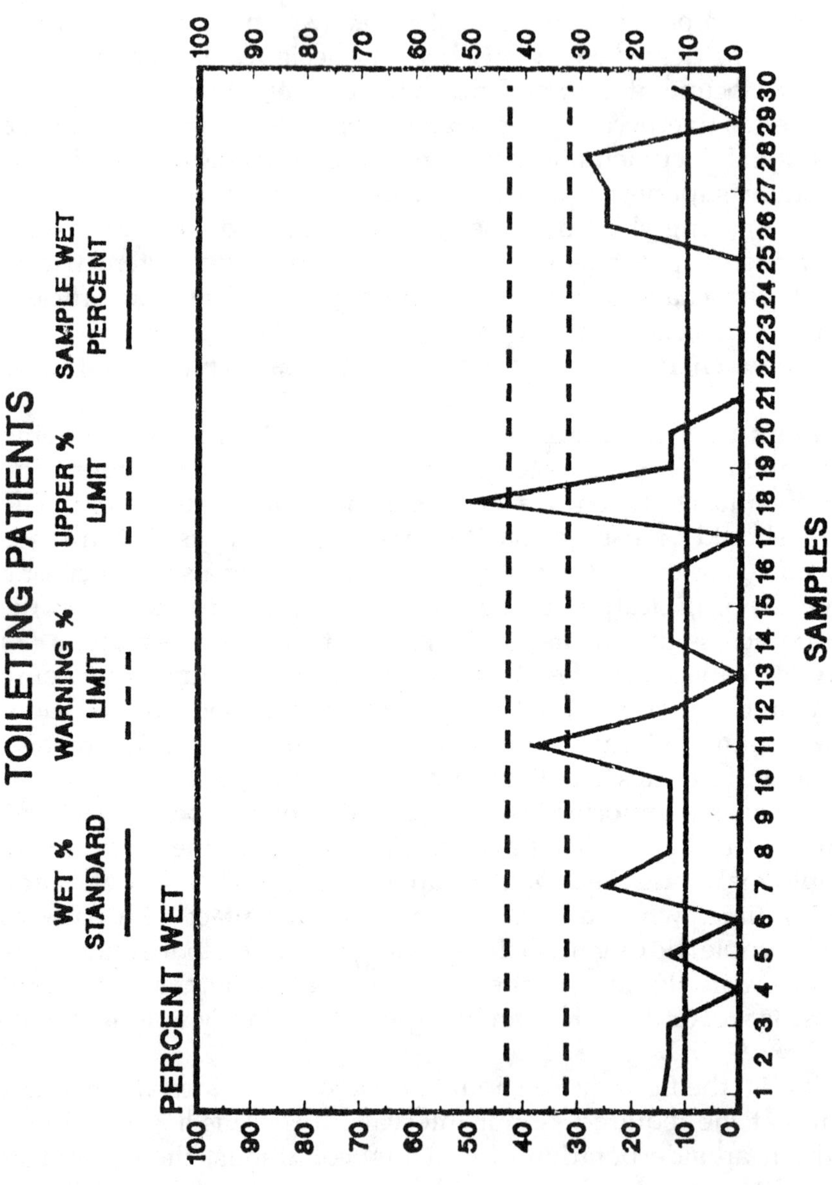

FIGURE 5.1 Example toileting chart.

results of patient checks in the supervisor check box. The specific role of the quality assurance nurse during the first program week is discussed in the next section.

The supervisor check is one of the active methods utilized to maintain the accuracy of aides' data recording. If supervisors use and pay attention to the charts, nurse's aides attribute more significance to data recording. The most inaccurate system is one in which aides see no visual evidence that supervisors attend to the information that is recorded. The documentation system recommended in this book corrects that problem. The frequency of floor-supervisor checks may be reduced after the first week. How to reduce the frequency of the checks is discussed in Chapter 8.

A second strategy used to make the charts active agents of management is to place them on clipboards that aides take to patients' rooms at the beginning of each shift. The boards are returned to the nurses' station within 15 minutes of the end of the shift. This system offers several advantages. First, it forces aides' attention on patients who are in the program. The behavioral act of "chart transport" required at the beginning of the shift reminds aides of what is to be done. Second, the chart-transport system brings aides into physical contact with patients at two critical times, the beginning and end of a shift. Thus, there is increased likelihood that patients will start and end a shift with a toileting opportunity.

Finally, the chart-transport system creates an opportunity for an aide–supervisor feedback session. Since charts are moved to the nurses' station at the end of each shift, the supervisor has a natural opportunity to review all charts and comment on patients' progress or aides' charting performance.

In summary, there are several points to be made about the documentation system. First, patient incontinence charts not only document patients' progress but also provide cues to manage nurse's aides' patient-care behavior. Second, incontinence charts work best if supervisors also use the charts. Third, charts should not be simply placed in patients' rooms and left there. They should be moved from the nurses' station to patients' rooms at shift beginning and ending. This transport system creates an opportunity for supervisor feedback and reminds aides when patients need toileting assistance. Aides and supervisors are now ready to be trained and the program started.

AIDE TRAINING

There are two major segments to aide training as it relates to incontinence care. Aides must be trained in basic job requirements and in the prompted-voiding protocol. This dual training can occur simultaneously.

The aide job-behavior checklist illustrated in Appendix C should be given to all aides at the beginning of the first shift on which the program is started. This checklist describes aides' major job requirements.

A supervisor should take a group of two to five aides through the checklist verbally and then walk through the steps with the aides. Supervisors can give the rationale of the steps to the aides while modeling the steps. For example, to model the first step, the supervisor should pick up the boards and take them to patients' rooms with the aides following along. The boards should be hung on prearranged hooks in patients' rooms. Next, supervisors can illustrate the prompted-voiding protocol.

Prior to modeling the prompted-voiding procedure, the supervisor should give aides the Prompted Voiding Checklist shown in Appendix C and the form shown in Figure 3.1 (Chapter 3) that illustrates the steps in prompted voiding. The nurse should tell aides to watch each step and to mark off the steps as they are shown. The supervisor then models the prompted voiding protocol and fills out the patient's chart based on the results of the prompts attempted. The group should then leave the room and review the prompted-voiding checklist verbally. This entire modeling–checklist process should be repeated with one more patient.

Aides should next be given an opportunity to conduct the procedures with a patient. The supervisor should fill out the checklist as each aide performs the prompted-voiding process and give immediate feedback about the aide's performance. This entire procedure should take approximately 30 to 60 minutes if three aides are trained. The modeling–checklist evaluation process is repeated each day until training is completed.

After all aides are trained, there should be two more brief evaluation sessions during the second week of the program. In these evaluation sessions a supervisor watches aides perform the prompted-voiding protocol and fills out the Prompted Voiding Checklist. The completed checklists are filed and used to document that aide floor training was completed.

Aides can easily learn the job performance required in the prompted-voiding protocol during the first program week. However, periodic reevaluations with the checklist (once per quarter) is probably a good idea. Such periodic reevaluations help fulfill requirements related to aide in-service training and should keep aides' attention on the key elements of the prompted-voiding protocol.

FLOOR SUPERVISOR TRAINING

Floor supervisors should accompany aides during the first training session and be exposed to the same training procedures. In addition, the Floor Supervisor Job Checklist (see Appendix C) should be given to each floor nurse after the initial training session with the aides.

The training supervisor should then walk the floor nurse through the checklist at some point during the first day. One complete round on all patients on a floor should provide adequate training.

The most important point to be learned during the floor nurse training session is how to check patients and how to note if a patient is wet (w) or dry (d) in the supervisor's block on the toileting documentation sheet (Figure 5.1). The floor nurse should also be trained to note if a chart is not filled out correctly. Floor supervisors should be able to learn the simple procedure in one brief training session. The Floor Supervisors Job Checklist listed in Appendix C should help the supervisor monitor the daily program mechanics.

QUALITY ASSURANCE NURSE

The quality assurance nurse must closely monitor all phases of the program during the first week. Checks on the program will be necessary two to three times per day. After the first week, the checks can be reduced significantly. Eventually, the quality assurance nurse can maintain the program with as little as one floor check per week.

The program start-up tasks of the quality assurance nurse are listed in Appendix C. These job requirements are designed to solve several major problems that typically occur when the program is instituted: forgetting, false-data recording, and poor checking.

Forgetting

Aides may have to be reminded several times during the first week to transport the toileting sheet forms to patients' rooms and to bring them back at the end of the shift. Also, there may be several instances in which patient charts are not filled out correctly. Most notably, there may be instances when there will not be chart entries for a 2-hour block.

It is the primary responsibility of the floor nurse to correct these charting problems. However, during the first week, the quality assurance nurse will have to conduct random checks and help correct charting errors. Experience indicates that floor nurses do not easily correct problems without support and feedback from professional supervisory nurses.

During the first week, the quality assurance nurse should check patients' rooms within 1 hour of the beginning of each shift and should also check at the nurses' station at the end of each shift. These checks should occur each day for 1 week and should prevent future problems with the transporting of charting boards. In addition, at the end of the shift the quality assurance nurse should make a quick review of the boards. This review should indicate if floor supervisors are entering information in the supervisor's block once per shift and if aides are charting correctly.

False Data Recording

False or inaccurate data recording is suspected if aides are recording unusually high levels of toileting or wet episodes. Since patients have been thoroughly assessed, the number of toileting and wet episodes expected of patients is known. These data are summarized in the final patient summary sheet described in Chapter 4. Patients selected for the toileting program should toilet no more than four times per day and should be wet no more than twice in a 12-hour period. Many patients will require only one or two toileting episodes per day and will not be wet at all.

The quality assurance nurse will know the number of toiletings and wet episodes expected of individual patients from patients' final assessment-data summary sheet (Chapter 4). Quick review of patients' charts during the first week as they are returned at the end of the shift will reveal instances in which unusually high wets or toiletings are recorded. For example, if a patient toilets only twice per day during the 6-day assessment period, but an aide records four toiletings and two wets, there is reason to believe that inaccurate recording is occurring. In these cases, responsible aides should be asked if they understand the system. In addition, the quality assurance nurse should alert aides to discrepancies between the patients' current records and patients' performance during the assessment period.

Poor Checking

Perhaps the most common error made by aides is to chart patients as dry when in fact they are wet. This error usually occurs either because the aide does not check the patient well or does not check the patient at all. In either case, a "dry" notation is made on the chart, and the patient remains wet.

The best way to correct this problem is time-consuming. It is necessary for the quality assurance nurse to mark the patient's linen with chalk and recheck the patient every 2 hours. If the patient is found wet and the linens are still marked, there is evidence that the aide did not do a good job of checking the patient for wetness. One or two patients for each aide can be marked daily during the first week to guard against this problem. Such intense, early supervision will prevent major future problems.

REDUCING SUPERVISION INTENSITY

Extensive floor supervision is required during the first week to fulfill training and management objectives. It is estimated that a quality assurance nurse will have to spend 2 to 3 hours per day for each of the first two shifts to start the program well. All staff should be trained and problems corrected at the end of this week. The daily suggested schedule and the responsibilities of quality assurance nurses and training nurses are listed in Appendix C ("Program Start-Up Tasks").

The steps described in the appendix are to be repeated exactly on Day 2 and Day 3. On Days 4 and 5 there should be no new aides to take on training rounds, and there should be no major problems to correct. Thus, the last 2 days are excellent times to refine the program. During these days the linen marking system discussed above can be implemented. The nurse should note if aides are marking patients as dry on the toileting chart during periods chalked wet linens are not changed. Feedback to aides when dry checks are being erroneously recorded should improve recording errors.

During the last 2 days aides could again be evaluated performing the prompted-voiding protocol and completing the Prompted Voiding Checklist. Excellent times for these evaluation checks are between 1:00 P.M. and 3:00 P.M. on the first shift and between 6:00 P.M. and 8:00 P.M. on the second shift.

Supervisory responsibilities are greatly reduced in the second week of the program. The quality assurance nurse need only make sure that patient charts are taken to the room at the beginning of each shift and returned at the end of the shift. The quality assurance nurse should begin a new and less intense quality-control system during this week. The specifics of the system are described in Chapter 6.

ADDING NEW PATIENTS

Newly admitted incontinent patients should be assessed as they enter the nursing home, and those who do well during the assessment period should be added to the toileting program. The addition of new patients is facilitated by the documentation system described in this chapter. Putting a patient's name on the toileting sheet, placing the clipboard at the nurses' station, and hanging a hook in the patient's room should start the patient on the program. The aide responsible for the patient should be alerted to the new clipboard that must be taken to the room. However, only a brief reminder should be necessary. All other program procedures remain the same.

The documentation and board-transport system described in this chapter are designed to focus aides' attention on toileting-program patients. If aides are confused about who is on the program, clipboards will be left at the nurses' station instead of moved to patients' rooms. The unmoved clipboards can be quickly detected by supervisors and the problem remedied. If the steps in this chapter are followed, the program should get off to a good start. It is now important to make sure the program is maintained at a high professional level. The quality-control system described in Chapter 6 should be implemented next.

Chapter 6

QUALITY CONTROL

What to learn from this chapter:

1. **The importance of quality control in preventing patient-care problems.**
2. **How to implement an incontinence quality-control system.**
3. **How to use quality-control information to identify problems in the incontinence-care process.**
4. **How to organize quality-control information to meet survey standards.**
5. **How to improve the patient-care process continuously with quality-control data.**

QUALITY CONTROL AND CONSISTENT PATIENT CONTACT

Several critical steps that provide the foundation for a successful incontinence program have been described. The division of patients into either toileting or changing protocols (Chapter 4) will assure that staff spend time toileting patients who can benefit from such time-consuming assistance. Implementing the staff training and program documentation procedures described in Chapter 5 should guarantee that staff know what to do. The next problem is to make sure the program continues to do well on a daily basis after it is successfully started. Program continuation is the subject of this chapter.

As stated earlier, one critical behavior is required of nurse's aides if patients are to be maintained in a dry state. The aides must contact patients on a 2-hour schedule and offer toileting assistance. If aides contact patients on a 4-hour schedule (miss one check), the probability that many patients will be found wet increases greatly. Thus, consistent and repetitive behavior (patient contact every 2 hours) is required 7 days a week.

Many factors influence the consistency of patient care. In the worst case, if the nursing home personnel situation deteriorates rapidly, consistent patient contact will rarely occur. Personnel crises can happen quickly as a result of the high proportion of untrained nursing aides and high staff turnover that characterizes nursing homes. This combination of factors produces a situation in which the loss of one or two good aides or floor supervisors leads to a quick and disastrous deterioration in patient care.

When consistent patient contact no longer occurs, the potential for general patient neglect and abuse increases. Patients will not get turned, hydrated, unrestrained, or toileted. To correct these problems, nurse managers must implement management systems that quickly signal staff inconsistency. A good information system prevents major problems and identifies factors that lead to patient-care problems. This type of information system is called a quality-control system. A major purpose of quality control is to maintain consistent levels of organizational performance, and quality-control systems can be easily applied to nursing staff behavior.

QUALITY-CONTROL PROCEDURES

A basic quality-control system has three major components: (1) standards of job performance must be defined, (2) job performance must be monitored and compared to these standards, and (3) methods to improve performance must be investigated when job standards are not met. In the best situation, quality control should not be used only to correct problems after they occur. Instead, a strategy of continuous improvement should be adopted.

To improve continously it is necessary to understand and identify all of the factors that lead to poor incontinence care. Such an understanding leads to continuous improvement in the work environment and to improvement in general patient care. Each of the three major points in a quality-control system—job standards, assessing job performance, and continuous improvement—is discussed separately in preparation to illustrating how a valid continence quality-control system can be implemented.

Job Performance Standards

Health care agencies often have difficulties in delineating job standards. For example, what are acceptable frequencies of skin breakdown in a facility, and how many patients must lose how much weight before patient-care quality is considered unacceptable? In addition, many patient-outcome measures used to define quality nursing performance cannot be linked directly to the daily care patients receive. Thus, nurse's aides can perform poorly—in terms of turning patients—for long periods before actual skin breakdown is obvious.

These factors limit the ability of quality-control systems to improve performance continuously. If problems are undetected for a long time, there is no good way to correct and improve job performance on a daily basis. This book describes a quality-control system that relies on more timely measures—measures that lead to continuous improvement.

The first step in this system is to set standards of how dry patients should be if they are toileted on a 2-hour schedule. These standards can be clearly defined following 6 days of assessment data. Once the dryness standards are known, the quality assurance nurse is ready to make rounds and collect data about the number of patients wet. Since job standards have been set, data collected are immediately interpretable. The quality assurance nurse can now move into job performance monitoring.

Job Performance Monitoring

Job performance monitoring of health care workers has been a particularly difficult problem. Aides perform most tasks in patients' rooms, out of view of supervisors. Poor job performance is often suspected only if patients suffer from unusual health problems. Excessive weight loss, skin breakdown, and high numbers of falls all indicate that nursing care is not good. However, identifying factors responsible for the problems is difficult, and more direct measures of actual patient-care behavior are often not available. A good system for monitoring job performance does not rely on "slow change" outcome measures. More direct and immediate information about job performance must be available.

The job performance monitoring system described in this book provides nurses with more immediate conclusions about the patient-care process. In fact, conclusions about whether patients are being toileted on a 2-hour schedule can be made immediately after each quality-control assessment.

The quality assurance nurse makes a round of all toileting patients and counts the number of patients found wet. After each round, the number of patients found wet can be compared to the job standard set during the assessment period. This comparison allows nurse managers to identify problems in the prompted-voiding program. If excessive numbers of patients are found wet after a round, immediate inquiries can be made into factors that may contribute to these problems.

Improving Performance

A good quality-control system will identify problems in patient care as they occur. What should happen once these problems are detected is another matter. Blaming poor employee performance for problems is the most typical managerial response. In addition, providing immediate job feedback to employees about problems often leads to quick improvement. This quick solution creates a sense of security that the problem has been well addressed. The employee feedback approach will work, and it is certainly better than doing nothing at all.

However, a more complete quality-control system attempts to identify all factors that contribute to poor patient-care performance. Is the problem always poorly motivated employees not doing what they are told? What other factors contribute to this poor motivation and poor performance? Are there work-scheduling difficulties or other problems with the work environment?

The quality-control system described in this book emphasizes an approach in which managers investigate multiple factors that contribute to poor incontinence care. Thus, the quality-control system should lead to an understanding of the total work environment as it relates to incontinence management. Making changes in the work environment based on valid quality-control data should lead to progressive and continued improvements in patient-care delivery. The next section describes how to apply the quality-control strategies.

TOILETING PROGRAM QUALITY CONTROL

Setting Job Standards

Two major descriptive statistics must be calculated to set job standards relevant to incontinence care. The average expected level of patients' wetness must be known, and how much this wetness will normally vary around the average must be calculated.

All job systems show some variability, and incontinence care is no exception. Because of unknown factors and factors beyond anyone's control, there will be variations in how many patients are found wet. Wetness variation will occur even if staff prompt and change patients on a consistent 2-hour schedule. The goal is to identify the normal or expected variability of patient wetness and to know when variability exceeds normal expectations.

The average number of patients expected to be wet and the expected variation around this average is set during the 6-day assessment period. During this period patients are prompted and checked every 2 hours. Thus, the level of patient dryness is established under conditions in which a consistent 2-hour schedule is in effect.

The average number of patients expected to be wet at any check and a variability estimate known as the standard deviation can be calculated from the 6 days of assessment data. The procedures for making this calculation are not difficult; they are reviewed in a stepwise fashion in Appendix D for those nurse managers who wish to learn them. Nurse managers with minimal statistical training should be able to follow these rules and calculate the average and standard deviation.

Once the average number of patients expected to be wet and the standard deviation is calculated from the assessment data, the nurse manager knows how many patients should be wet if they are prompted on a 2-hour schedule. In general, the percentage of patients wet at any given hour should be within the average or within two standard deviations from the average. If the number found wet is more than two standard deviations from the average, you should suspect that the continence-care system is not doing well. If the number wet is more than three standard deviations from the average, the incontinence program has problems.

The entire matter of statistical calculation can be handled more simply for those nurse managers not wanting to get involved in calculating standard deviations. Since only patients with appropriate toileting rates above 66% will be included in the program, the following rules hold true. First, at any given hour the percentage of toileting-program patients found wet should be between 10% and 20%. Second, if 40% of the patients are found wet, problems with the incontinence care system should be suspected. Third, if 50% or more of the patients are found wet, major problems have developed, and it is likely that aides are not implementing prompted voiding on the 2-hour schedule. For example, if 4 patients out of 10 (40%) are found wet, there is reason to believe problems are occurring. The nurse manager should alert the floor nurse to the problem and instruct her or him to make certain that patients are dry and toileted. If 5 or more patients out of 10 are found wet (50%), major problems have developed, and steps should be taken to correct the problem. Inquiries as to how this problem developed should be made.

Job Performance Monitoring

The quality assurance nurse monitors performance of the toileting program by making a round of all toileting-program patients. The form illustrated in Figure 6.1 is used to collect job performance information. Two major types of data are collected: (1) data con-

B & B QUALITY ASSURANCE FORM

Attends® Caring Practices

Date: ________ Time: ________ Your Name/Title: ______________________ Su M T W Th F S (circle)

			Nurse Assistant Errors (X)					Supervisor Errors (X)				
Resident's Name	(X) Wet	(X) Dry	No Chart	N.A. Name Missing	Check Missing or Incomplete	Resident Name Missing	Full Form	Unmarked N.A. Error	Check Missing	Time/Initials Missing	Total # Errors	Last Void (Time)
		X										
		X										
		X										
		X										
		X										
		X										
		X										
		X										
	X				X			X			2	
		X										

RESULTS:
1. Overall # of residents checked 10
2. Overall # of residents found dry 9
3. Overall # of residents found wet 1
4. % of residents wet on this check (divide #3 by #1) 10%
5. % of residents dry on this check (divide #2 by #1) 90%

FIGURE 6.1 Quality assurance form.

cerning patient continence condition (dry/D or wet/W) and (2) job performance data relating to how well the toileting charts are being completed. A round of 10 patients should take approximately 15 minutes if the nurse fills out only the quality assurance form.

Each patient is checked for wetness or dryness, and a notation is made about their condition (the first two columns on the form). The incontinence chart for each patient is quickly reviewed while the nurse is in the patient's room, and notations are made of any errors. Common aide errors include the following:

1. Chart not hung in patient's room ("No Chart" column on form).
2. Nurse's aide's name not listed on chart ("N.A. Name Missing" column) or date missing.
3. A 2-hour block with no information entered about a patient's incontinence condition ("Check missing or Incomplete" column).
4. Resident's name missing on the chart ("Resident Name Missing" column).
5. Toileting form is completely filled out and not replaced with a new form ("Full Form" column).

Floor supervisors also have a role in the incontinence charting and should be held responsible for overall quality of the chart. Common supervisor errors that should be monitored by the quality assurance nurse are as follows:

1. Aide errors are not noted by the supervisor nurse. The floor nurse is to check the charts to make notes if aide errors have occurred. If any aide charting errors are present without a note by a supervisor on the chart, an unmarked error should be recorded under "Supervisor Errors" ("Unmarked N.A. Error" column).

2. The supervisor is responsible for checking the patient once per shift and noting if the patient is wet or dry. The time of the check and the supervisor's initials should appear in the supervisor block on the toileting sheet. A supervisor error is noted if a chart does not have a supervisor check ("Check Missing" column) or if the supervisor's initials are missing ("Time/Initials missing").

3. The last column on the quality-assessment chart is optional. The last time the patient voided is recorded (continent or incontinent). If a very long time has elapsed since the last patient void was noted (6 hours or more), one may suspect problems with either the patient (i.e., urinary retention) or the accuracy of aide recording.

All errors found on the board should be noted on the quality-control form. In addition, a written message should be placed on the toileting chart, asking the responsible aide or supervisory nurse to correct the error. Once the round is complete, the quality assurance nurse quickly summarizes the data and chooses one of the quality assurance response alternatives listed on the back of the Quality Assurance Form. These response alternatives are listed in Figure 6.2

It is important to remember that these responses are simply meant to give objective feedback to employees about the results of the quality assurance check. Employees should not be blamed at this point if there is an unusually high number of patients found wet (responses 2 or 3). If high numbers of patients are found wet, floor nurses and other employees should be interviewed in an effort to determine the reason for the problem. Such cooperative involvement of employees and quality assurance nurses should eventually lead to the identification of problems and to improvements in employee motivation.

The Quality Assurance Form (Figure 6.1) illustrates the case in which only 1 patient out of 10 was found wet. Thus, a variation of response alternative 1 (Figure 6.2) was chosen. There was a 2-hour interval in which no notation was made on the patient's chart, and the supervisor did not catch this error. Thus, a nurse-assistant error (Check Missing column) and a supervisor error ("Unmarked N.A. Error") was noted for this patient.

Improving Performance

The quality-control system described to this point will at least prevent major or chronic problems from developing in the toileting program. Quick detection of instances when an excessive number of patients are wet reduces the chance of patient neglect.

Continually improving the system, however, requires more analytical efforts. It is necessary to compare times when the quality-control data are good to the times when they are bad. Such comparison leads to an understanding of how the work environment contributes to problems in the incontinence system.

The form illustrated in Figure 6.3 is one method of making such

Instructions

After completing each Quality Assurance form, use the appropriate response listed below to give your charge nurses positive or negative feedback. They in turn respond appropriately to the nurse assistants.

CONDITION OF RESIDENTS ON ANY ONE B&B QUALITY ASSURANCE CHECK:

1. 0 or 1 Resident Wet on Each Hall:

Response: (choose one)

A. You are doing a good job with the incontinent program residents. Keep up the good work. This is the condition we should always keep these residents in. Thank you.

B. The incontinent program residents were recently checked, and they were found to be dry. Thanks. This indicates we have all been doing well with these residents. Thanks again, and let's stay on the job.

C. We are keeping the program residents continent. Good job. Thanks for your cooperation and hard work.

2. 2 Residents Wet on Each Hall:

Response: (choose one)

A. We need to attend to the incontinent program residents more closely than we are presently. So let's try harder to keep these residents dry.

B. We can do a better job working with the incontinent program residents. We are slipping, so let's get back on the job.

3. 3 or More Residents Wet on Each Hall:

Response: (choose one)

A. The incontinent program residents are entirely too wet. There is no reason for this number of residents to be wet at any one time. Let's go and check these residents, change the ones who are wet and offer assistance to toilet to all of these residents now. Report back to me which residents appropriately toileted.

B. Concerning the incontinent program residents, we have not been doing as we were asked to do. We know what is expected of us, so let's go now and check these residents, change the ones who are wet and offer toileting assistance to all of them. Report back on which residents appropriately toileted.

(Note: If 3 or more residents continue to be wet on your checks you may need to review the B&B video and procedures with the staff and/or the resident's status.)

FIGURE 6.2 Quality assurance response list.

Time	Mon.	Tues.	Wed.	Thur.	Fri.	Sat.	Sun.
8							
9							
10							
11							
12							
2							
3							
3							
4							
5							
6							
7							
8							
9							

Personnel

- Work Short Part of Shift
- Work Short Entire Shift
- New Aide on Floor
- New Supervisor on Floor
- Other

Patient

- Patient Sick
- Excessive Bowel Movement Noted
- Patient Relocated
- Medicine Change on Patient

Incontinence Procedures

- Board Not in Patient's Room
- 2-Hour Time Blocks on Chart With No Entry
- Supervisor Checks Missing
- Other Board Errors

FIGURE 6.3 Fishbone chart.

an analysis. This type of chart is called a fishbone chart by quality-control professionals.

Patterns may emerge from the fishbone chart that reveal work or environmental factors that contribute to problems. One simply writes on the chart the conditions that existed when a quality-control round revealed an excessive number of patients wet. Critical areas that could explain a bad work sample are listed on the vertical lines. In this case, personnel, incontinence procedures, time of day, and patients are the major areas that could produce problems.

Thus, if a quality assurance nurse samples patients on Monday at 8:00 A.M. and finds a large number wet, she or he should enter the percentage found wet on the 8/Monday line in the fishbone chart. In addition, the nurse should note other factors present at that time. Thus, if boards were found missing from patients' rooms, indicating that aides were not implementing the incontinence procedures, a notation of the time and day should be placed under the appropriate incontinence procedure error column.

The following example from a nursing home setting illustrates how this process can work. In this nursing home there was a large number of samples in which patients were found excessively wet at 12:00 P.M. An investigation into this time period revealed that aides on one floor had an unusually large number of patients who required feeding assistance. The time consumed by this feeding made it difficult for aides to check toileting-program patients before 1:00 P.M. Unfortunately, at 1:00 P.M., half of the aides left on break. Thus, the full staff was not available for incontinence care until 1:30 P.M.

The problem was resolved by having a volunteer worker assist with feeding between 11:00 A.M. and 1:00 P.M. The volunteer worker freed nurse's aides to do incontinence care. This example illustrates how a good quality-control program should work. A good system not only prevents problems but suggests solutions that produce continuous improvement in the work environment. Such improvements reduce the number of times that a sample of patients will be found unusually wet. Improvement of the incontinence system should continue until eventually the system will work with only minimal effort by managers.

Display of Job Data-Control Charts

To illustrate trends, patterns, and general variability in job performance as it affects patient wetness, it is typical to use a control chart. A sample control chart for one nursing home is illustrated in Figure 6.4. In this control chart, the percentage of patient wetness is listed on the vertical line of the graph, and successive samples are listed on the horizontal line. The average expected level of patient wetness, as determined by assessment data, is indicated by a solid horizontal line. Broken lines indicate points at two standard deviations and three standard deviations above this average.

Resident's Name ______________________ Room # __________

Instructions: Place an X through the correct symbol(s) each time you check the resident.

little wet	or	very wet	or	dry

Toileted ____cc (amount)	BM bowel movement	takes drink

TWO DAY SUMMARY	
1. # Supervisory Cks	____
2. # Dry	____
3. Percent Dry	____

Date ______________________

Nurse Asst. Name ______________________

Time	little wet	very wet	dry	Toileted	BM	takes drink
7 AM				____cc	BM	____cc
8				____cc	BM	____cc
9				____cc	BM	____cc
10				____cc	BM	____cc
11				____cc	BM	____cc
12 PM				____cc	BM	____cc
1				____cc	BM	____cc
2				____cc	BM	____cc

Supv. Initials/Time: ____/____ ____/____ ____/____

Nurse Asst. Name ______________________

Time	little wet	very wet	dry	Toileted	BM	takes drink
3 PM				____cc	BM	____cc
4				____cc	BM	____cc
5				____cc	BM	____cc
6				____cc	BM	____cc
7				____cc	BM	____cc
8				____cc	BM	____cc
9				____cc	BM	____cc
10				____cc	BM	____cc

Supv. Initials/Time: ____/____ ____/____ ____/____

Nurse Asst. Name ______________________

Time	little wet	very wet	dry	Toileted	BM	takes drink
11 PM				____cc	BM	____cc
12 AM				____cc	BM	____cc
1				____cc	BM	____cc
2				____cc	BM	____cc
3				____cc	BM	____cc
4				____cc	BM	____cc
5				____cc	BM	____cc
6				____cc	BM	____cc

Supv. Initials/Time: ____/____ ____/____ ____/____

	# Wet Checks	# Dry Checks	# Dry Runs to toilet	# Voided in toilet
s				

Date ______________________

Nurse Asst. Name ______________________

Time	little wet	very wet	dry	Toileted	BM	takes drink
7 AM				____cc	BM	____cc
8				____cc	BM	____cc
9				____cc	BM	____cc
10				____cc	BM	____cc
11				____cc	BM	____cc
12 PM				____cc	BM	____cc
1				____cc	BM	____cc
2				____cc	BM	____cc

Supv. Initials/Time: ____/____ ____/____ ____/____

Nurse Asst. Name ______________________

Time	little wet	very wet	dry	Toileted	BM	takes drink
3 PM				____cc	BM	____cc
4				____cc	BM	____cc
5				____cc	BM	____cc
6				____cc	BM	____cc
7				____cc	BM	____cc
8				____cc	BM	____cc
9				____cc	BM	____cc
10				____cc	BM	____cc

Supv. Initials/Time: ____/____ ____/____ ____/____

Nurse Asst. Name ______________________

Time	little wet	very wet	dry	Toileted	BM	takes drink
11 PM				____cc	BM	____cc
12 AM				____cc	BM	____cc
1				____cc	BM	____cc
2				____cc	BM	____cc
3				____cc	BM	____cc
4				____cc	BM	____cc
5				____cc	BM	____cc
6				____cc	BM	____cc

Supv. Initials/Time: ____/____ ____/____ ____/____

	# Wet Checks	# Dry Checks	# Dry Runs to toilet	# Voided in toilet
Totals				

FIGURE 6.4 Data-control chart.

Once the chart is made, the quality assurance nurse simply graphs the percentage of patients found wet on each quality assurance round. For example, in Figure 6.4 the first four samples reveal the following percentages of patients wet: 15%, 12%, 0%, 12%. Samples above the warning limit were not observed until the 18th round, in which 48% of the patients were wet.

Employees are often taught to read control charts, and the charts can be placed in an area where they are visible to employees at the nurses' station. Control charts can serve as a constant reminder of job performance. In the best situation, employees will be stimulated by the control chart to offer suggestions that will improve the incontinence work situation. A control chart useful for monitoring toileting-program patients is reproduced in Appendix D. Control limits and average job-performance standards that should apply to most nursing home toileting patients are already noted on this chart.

Control charts are a useful addition to the incontinence quality-control program, and constructing control charts is not difficult. If the nursing home does not calculate standard deviations, the control chart can still be constructed on the basis of the suggested standard figures: 40% wet indicates a potential problem, and 50% wet indicates a severe problem.

Despite the potential value and visual appeal of control charts, their use is optional for the quality-control programs described in this book. It is possible to maintain the incontinence program at a high professional level and even make continuing program improvements without graphing. If nurse managers find the charts difficult to construct or understand, they should not be used.

There are computer software programs available that organize all quality-control data and perform all technical operations described in this chapter, including calculating standard deviations and constructing fully operational control charts. These programs work on most personal computers.

QUALITY CONTROL AND CHANGE PATIENTS

Approximately 50% of patients, because of their inability to store urine or to control the voiding process, will not be on a toileting program. These patients are best managed with the check–change protocol described in chapter 3. In almost all cases it is necessary to check and change these patients every 2 hours throughout the 7:00 A.M. to 9:00 P.M. period. Such a check–change schedule will not keep these patients dry, but it will minimize how long and how much they are wet.

Unfortunately, check–change patients are easy to ignore. Typically, they are more debilitated than patients on the toileting program. This debilitation often means that the patients are very unresponsive and generally uncomplaining about their care. This combination of circumstances increases the importance of implementing a quality-control program that facilitates consistent staff implementation of the check–change procedures.

Unfortunately, the quality-control system for check–change patients is more difficult to develop and implement than the toileting quality-control system. Because of these difficulties, nurse managers should probably concentrate first on implementing a quality-control system for the toileting program. Once the toileting program is implemented, the more challenging and time-consuming check–change quality-control systems can be attempted. This is discussed in the following section, which is organized within the same quality-control framework used to discuss toileting patients. This format involves a discussion of setting job standards, job performance monitoring, and continuous improvement.

Job Standards

The primary information used to control the quality of the toileting program is the number of patients found wet on any round. This wet-frequency information is usable because most toileting patients should be dry most of the time if the prompted-voiding protocol is conducted consistently. Thus, large numbers of wet patients signify that something unusual is happening.

Unfortunately, the same wetness-frequency information is not as usable for check–change patients. Check–change patients have higher frequencies of incontinence than do toileting patients. This higher frequency means that most check–change patients will be found wet on a round even if staff implement the protocol on a consistent 2-hour schedule. In other words, even if a nurse manager samples 10 check–change protocol patients and finds all of them wet (100%), it will still not be possible to conclude that problems exist with the check–change care system.

Because of these problems it is necessary to use incontinence volumes as the primary control measure—the volume measures that were collected during the assessment period and were summarized in the final assessment-data form (Chapter 4). A final assessment-data form for a typical check–change program patient is reproduced in Figure 6.5.

The expected or average job standard for use with check–change patients is the average incontinence volume that resulted from 6 days of implementing the check–change protocol every 2 hours. Thus, in the case of the check–change patient assessed in Figure 6.5 the average incontinence volume is 100 cc. This means that if the patient's pads are found wet on any round, the volume of wetness in those pads should be around 100 cc.

The standard deviation of the expected wetness volumes can also be calculated to describe the variability in the expected wet volumes of the patients changed every 2 hours. Thus, as with the toileting patients, wetness volumes that exceed expected levels can be set at two or three standard deviations above the average. A step-by-step description of how to calculate this type of standard deviation appears in Appendix D.

More simply, the quality assurance nurse could use the average expected volumes and the highest incontinence volume observed during the assessment period as job standards. The highest volume listed in the summary sheet for the sample patient (Figure 6.5) was 250 cc. Thus, if a pad is weighed and found to contain a higher wetness volume than 250 cc, you might conclude that potential problems are developing.

The check–change control chart illustrated in Figure 6.6 can be used to monitor the change process. The "Pad Dry Wgt." column refers to the dry weight for the type of pad the patient is wearing. Pad preweights can be calculated by weighing 20 to 25 of each type of pad the nursing home uses and averaging the weights of these pads. Thus, the average weight of a disposable pad may be 120 g, and the average dry weight of a reusable laundry pad might be 300 g.

The nurse simply checks the patient, notes the type of pad, and

Patient's Name ______________
Date ______________

Final Assessment Summary Sheet and Treatment Decision

Toileting Ability

Appropriate Toileting %	Check Appr. Box
0%–65% Poor ability to toilet	X
66%–75% Average ability to toilet	
75%–100% Excellent ability to toilet	

Bladder Storage Ability

Frequency of wets per day:

0–1 Good ability to prevent incontinence	
1–2 Marginal ability to prevent incontinence	
2+ Poor ability to prevent incontinence	X

Volume of wets per day:

0–30 cc Good ability to control urine loss	
30–75 cc Marginal ability to control urine loss	
75+ cc Poor ability to control urine loss	X

Mental Responsiveness

No question answered—poor responsiveness	X
Answered 50% correctly—marginal responsiveness	
Answered 75% correctly—excellent responsiveness	

6-Day Assessment Summary

Toileting ability

Column
1 total no. wets 15
2 total no. toilets 1
3 total no. voids (columns 1 + 2) 16
4 % appr. toilet $\frac{\text{(column 2)}}{\text{(column 3)}}$ $\frac{1}{16} = .06$

Storage ability

5 No. expected wets per day $\frac{\text{(total wets)}}{6} = \frac{15}{6} = 2.5$

6 Avg. vol. inc. episodes $\frac{\text{(add all inc. vols)}}{\text{(column 1)}} = \frac{1500}{15} = 100$

7 Lowest inc. vol 25
Largest Inc. vol 250

Responsiveness

Column
8 no. yes correct responses 4
9% correct $\frac{\text{(col. 8)}}{\text{no. days in prompted voiding} \times 6} = \frac{4}{36} = 11\%$

FIGURE 6.5 Final assessment chart.

Dry Weights of Pads

Blue 25 Green 275
Red 15 White 250

Patient name	Pad dry wgt.	Pad wet wgt.	Diff. wet vol.	Exp. wet	Warning wet	Checks in control out control	Patient position	Skin wet red OK
Smith	250	400	150	100	200	IN	SIDE	OK

FIGURE 6.6 Wetness volume control chart.

enters the average dry weight that has been precalculated for that type of pad. If the pad is wet when it is checked, it should be placed in a small garbage bag and replaced with a dry pad. When the quality assurance nurse returns to her office, the garbage bag is weighed and the pad weight entered. The difference in weight between the dry pad and the wet pad provides an excellent estimate of the volume of patient wetness.

Finally, the quality assurance nurse enters the difference in pad weights in the "Diff. Wet Vol." column and indicates if the wet volume is in the expected wet range ("Exp. Wet" column) or beyond expected range ("Warning Wet" column) above two standard deviations or above highest wet volume. Remember, each patient will have a different standard. If the pad weight exceeds that standard, the nurse should immediately ask the aide responsible for the patient about potential problems. If the volume is in the expected or normal range, aides should be informed that the patient is doing well and that the 2-hour check–change system is in control.

The last two columns in the table are optional, but they can provide useful information about the patient's condition. If the patient is on a turning program, his or her position (back, side, etc.) can be noted. The patient's skin condition can also be noted in terms of its wetness or redness. If there are no problems, a simple "OK" can be entered in the last column.

The numbers in Figure 6.6 represent a check on a sample patient whose data are shown in the final assessment form. The patient was wearing a white reusable pad. The nurse entered the average weight of the pad in the dry pad weight column as 250. The patient was found wet, and the pad was found to weigh 400 g. The difference in the dry and wet weight was 150 g. The expected wetness volume of this patient as calculated from the assessment period was 100 cc. The highest wetness volume, which signifies a problem, was in the 250-cc range. The sample wetness volumes of this patient (150) is between the expected wetness (100) and the control limit (250). Thus, the patient is said to be "in control." The patient was found in a "side" position, and the skin was judged to be "OK." The conclusion is made that the check–change process for this patient is working well.

Since individual job standards are set for each patient, the quality assurance nurse need not check all patients. In fact, completely sampling pad weights of all patients on any one round would prove excessively time-consuming. In normal circumstances the quality assurance nurse should probably check only one patient for each aide working. This sampling should provide adequate information about how the check–change protocol is being administered throughout the facility. If one patient or the patients of one aide produced successive high wet-volume samples, that would justify more intense sampling of that aide or patient.

Continuous Improvement

The same continuous-improvement management strategy used with toileting-control patients should also apply to the check–change quality-control system. In fact, the same fishbone problem chart used to identify factors that contribute to high wet frequency in toileting patients can be used to analyze unusually high wet volumes. Continued analysis of instances in which patients are found exceptionally wet should lead to information about factors in the work environment that contribute to high wet volumes and eventually should reduce the variability of the wet pad weights. The work environment will continue to improve, and patient neglect resulting from inconsistent aide behavior will be reduced dramatically.

Chapter 7

NIGHT INCONTINENCE CARE

What to learn from this chapter:

1. **How to individualize nighttime incontinence programs.**
2. **Why daytime toileting schedules should not be individualized.**
3. **How to assess patients for individualized nighttime incontinence care.**
4. **How to control the quality of nighttime incontinence programs.**

INDIVIDUALIZATION OF PATIENT CHECKING SCHEDULES

The previous chapters have made the case that incontinent patients should be checked every 2 hours from 7:00 A.M. to 9:00 P.M. Either the prompted-voiding or check–change protocol should be implemented during this period to keep patients in an optimally dry condition.

Many toileting-program patients could be kept dry with a checking schedule of 3 or even 4 hours. These patients can be identified in several ways: (a) they will always be found dry during the quality assurance nurse's control-check rounds, (b) they will be charted as voiding only two or three times per day by the aides, and (c) they will always answer the question "Are you wet or dry?" accurately. Time could be saved by individualizing the checking schedule for the latter patients. However, such individualization is probably not worth the problems it would cause during the waking hours of approximately 7:00 A.M. to 9:00 P.M.

Serious management problems arise when staff have to remember different patient schedules. It is easy to miss a round on the patient with an unusual 3- or 4-hour checking schedule when the majority of patients are on a 2-hour schedule. The result of missing even one 3-hour check means that a patient will have to wait 6 or more hours for toileting assistance. In addition, even if patients do not require toileting assistance every 2 hours, they still benefit from the social stimulation of a 2-hour staff-contact schedule. There are a variety of reasons that individualizing schedules from 7:00 A.M. to 9:00 P.M. is not recommended.

This recommendation changes for the 9 P.M. to 6:00 A.M. period. Efforts should be made during this normal sleep period to be minimally disruptive to a patient's sleep. Sleep disruption can be particularly minimized for those patients who do not require a 2-hour check.

To understand how to design a nighttime incontinence program, nurse managers must understand three basic nursing issues: (1) what is known about a patient's sleep patterns, (2) who can be safely checked on a 3-hour-plus schedule, and (3) what is known about nighttime incontinence and how it influences individualized schedules.

SLEEP

Sleep patterns change with age. One of the most notable changes is that for elderly people sleep becomes "fragmented." Fragmented sleep means that patients do not sleep for long periods. Instead, they sleep for shorter periods with intervals of wakefulness between the sleep periods. This problem is particularly severe for nursing home patients.

Nursing home patients have been reported to sleep only an average of 13.5 minutes per hour. Observations indicate that few patients sleep a complete hour even during the peak sleep periods from 6:00 P.M. to 8:00 A.M. Overall, nursing home patients sleep an average of 8 hours per day but attain these sleep hours by spending long periods of time in bed (Ancoli-Israel, Parker, Sinaee, Fell, & Kripke, 1989).

The specific factors that contribute to sleep fragmentation are not well known. Some people identify excessive noise, bright lights, and poor temperature regulation as contributing to sleep problems. Because of natural changes in sleep patterns the elderly may be more sensitive to such environmental disruption.

Other people argue that nursing staff routines may unnecessarily disrupt patients. Checking patients every 2 hours all night would seem to be particularly disruptive to sleep. In fact, preliminary indications suggest that patients do wake a majority of the time during the process of the nighttime check. They often wake even if they are not changed or repositioned. Are such checks necessary? Do the advantages of such a checking schedule justify potential side effects resulting from patients' sleep deprivation?

WHO CAN SAFELY BE CHECKED ON A 3-HOUR SCHEDULE

Patients are often checked every 2 hours throughout the night to prevent skin breakdown. Repositioning the patient or changing wet bed linens are the primary preventive-care activities.

The risk for skin ulceration increases with age and immobility. Thus, nursing home patients are a primary at-risk population. Incontinent nursing home patients, who are more physically debilitated than continent patients, are a particularly high-risk group.

Numerous factors have been identified as increasing the risk for skin problems. Physiological factors include over- or underweight, poor nutrition, and poor hydration. Environmental factors include excessive skin moisture or dryness and the abrasiveness of padding. Physical factors include prolonged pressure on bony prominences. The pressure factor has provided the primary justification for turning patients on a 2-hour schedule. A 2-hour or even more frequent turning schedule seems justified for all patients who show risk factors for skin ulceration. Alternatively, less frequent turning or checking schedules are probably justified for some low-risk patients.

The skin breakdown potential of patients can be evaluated in several ways. One standardized evaluation instrument to assess skin breakdown risk is a Norton index. The Norton index rates patients on a 4-point scale in five major areas: physical condition, mental status, activity, mobility, and incontinence. The lower the score, the higher the risk, with a score of 14 being the conventional cutoff. Patients scoring below 14 are at a high risk for decubitus ulcer development. Because of this risk, all incontinent patients with Norton scores below 14 probably need to be checked on a 2-hour schedule throughout the 24-hour period. Patients with a score above 14 are candidates for a less frequent nighttime check–change schedule. This less frequent scheduling is particularly justified if the check disrupts the patient's sleep.

NIGHTTIME INCONTINENCE

Preliminary indications suggest that nursing home patients void about as frequently during the night as they do during the day (O'Donnell, Beck, & Walls, 1990). There is conflicting evidence, however, about the volume of the nighttime voids. Even if nighttime output is higher than during the day, there are still many patients whose night output is so low that it could be easily absorbed by most padding systems. In fact, some padding systems have been evaluated that hold as many as three seperate patient voids before skin wetness can be detected (Sowell, Schnelle, Hu, & Traughber, 1987).

The presence of effective absorbent systems means that many incontinent patients do not need to be checked and changed on a 2-hour schedule throughout the night. Patients whose incontinence volumes over a 3-hour period could be safely contained are candidates for an individualized nighttime incontinence-care program. A 3- or even 4-hour checking and changing program would be adequate to manage the nighttime incontinence of these patients safely. The trick is to identify patients whose incontinence patterns and skin ulceration risk would justify an individualized nighttime changing schedule. The advantage of such a schedule may be a higher-quality nighttime sleeping environment.

There are two major issues in designing a nighttime incontinence program. First, patients who can safely be placed on an individual nighttime checking schedule must be identified. This is an assessment issue. Second, a method to assure quality control for the nighttime program must be implemented.

ASSESSMENT

Two assessment criteria are used to identify the type of patient who is a candidate for an individualized nighttime incontinence program. The patient's skin condition must tolerate a 3-hour-plus turning or repositioning schedule, and the patient's incontinence volume should not exceed the absorbent capacity of the incontinence pads. There are two stages to the assessment process: an initial patient screen and, for patients who pass the screen, a 6-night assessment process that tests the validity of the screen.

The screen primarily involves an evaluation of the patient's risk for skin breakdown. Many nursing homes already use some method to evaluate which patients are at risk for pressure-sore development so that turning schedules can be planned. Patients identified as at lower risk for development of decubitus ulcers could be included in the more intense weeklong assessment process.

If nursing homes do not currently utilize a skin risk evaluation system, the Norton index could be used. A complete description of how to rate a patient on the Norton index appears in several of the references listed at the end of this chapter. Patients scoring above 14 on the Norton index possibly do not need to be turned on a 2-hour schedule throughout the night (Goldstein & Goldstein 1982; Taylor, 1988).

If a patient's status is questionable, direct observations should be made of the patient's ability to turn himself or herself. A patient could be placed in one body position (left side) and observations made at 2-hour intervals. If the patient independently changes position, he or she is a candidate for the 3-hour-plus turning program. These behavioral observations of patients' turning ability could be completed during daytime hours when the patient is in bed. Once the screen is completed, a more comprehensive assessment takes place over 6 days. The steps in this 6-day patient assessment are listed in Figure 7.1.

All patients who pass the screen should be checked on a 3-hour schedule starting at 9:00 P.M. Thus, the patient is checked at 9:00 P.M., midnight, 3:00 A.M., and 6:00 A.M. A nighttime assessment sheet should be utilized to facilitate completion of this checking schedule. This form is identical to the daytime assessment form with the exception of the 3-hour checking interval. Patients on the daytime toileting program can be prompted during the 3-hour nighttime checks if they are awake. Patients on the daytime check–change program should continue to be changed at night. Thus, the daytime check–change patients will not be asked the wet–dry question and will be toileted only if they request assistance. Figure 7.2 illustrates the nighttime assessment sheet for a hypothetical patient.

All incontinent patients should be placed on a padding system that is advertised to be absorbent. Wet patients should be changed at 3-hour intervals and the absorbent pads placed in small garbage bags. The pads are taken to the nurses' station at the end of the round and given to the supervisory nurse for weighing.

The quality assurance nurse should make two successive rounds with each aide during the first 2 nights for all 3-hour schedule patients. The quality assurance nurse can train the night aides in either the prompted-voiding or the check–change pro-

1. Check patients at 9:00 P.M., midnight 3 A.M., and 6:00 A.M.
2. Use a nighttime assessment sheet and do the same protocol (prompted-void or check–change) that the patient is on during the day.
3. Place each wet pad in a garbage bag and take to the nurses' station for weighing.
4. Quality assurance nurse makes trwo successive rounds with each aide for each 3-hour patient. Checks are made for skin wetness, redness, and urine output. Use the daytime quality-control sheet for the check–change program used.
5. Daytime nurse checks patients' skin at the end of the first week.
6. Data are summarized on the nighttime assessment-data sheet, and a determination is made about the patient's schedule of nighttime checks. Average expected level of wetness and control limits are set for the 3-hour-schedule patients.

FIGURE 7.1 Nighttime assessment checklist.

Patient Name Smith
Nurse's Name Brown
Date ______

Checks	Wetness		Toilet		Responsiveness			Volume	
	Patient was		Did pat. toilet		Did patient answer question wet or dry			Volume of voids	
7:00 P.M.	wet	dry	yes	no	yes correct	yes incorrect	no answer	cont	incon 125
9:00 P.M.	wet	dry	yes	no	yes correct	yes incorrect	no answer	cont	incon
12:00 A.M.	wet	dry	yes	no	yes correct	yes incorrect	no answer	cont	incon
3:00 A.M.	wet	dry	yes	no	yes correct	yes incorrect	no answer	cont	incon 135
6:00 A.M.	wet	dry	yes	no	yes correct	yes incorrect	no answer	cont	incon 150

Summary	No. of wets	No. toilets	No. correct	No. incorrect	No	No. cont.	volume incon
	3	0	5	0	0	0	410

$$\frac{0}{3 + 0} = 0\ \%\ \text{Appropriate toileting}$$

Decision Point:

There is no decision. Continue assessment for 6 nights unless there are changes in skin health.

FIGURE 7.2 Nightime assessment sheet.

tocol during these rounds. The same modeling–checklist training procedure used during the day can be utilized at night.

More important, the patient's skin should be checked during each round by the quality assurance nurse. If the patient's skin feels wet or if excessive redness is found, a notation is made on the same data sheet used to monitor the daytime check–change program (Figure 6.6, Chapter 6). The patient should be repositioned and the position noted.

During the next round, patients are again checked, and all relevant information is recorded, including patients' body positions. It is particularly noteworthy if the patient has changed position from one round to the next. Patients who independently change positions do not need to be turned on a 2-hour schedule. Finally, at the end of the first week, the daytime nurse should independently evaluate patients' skin conditions.

All assessment data should be summarized at the end of the first week and a second decision made about all patients. Those who show either skin irritation or excessive skin wetness on the 3-hour checking rounds should be returned to a 2-hour schedule. Patients who show no skin irritation or minimal wetness can be started on the 3-hour schedule. A good general rule is that if the patient has no 3-hour volumes over 250 cc and averages less than one bowel movement per night, that patient can be safely managed on a 3-hour schedule with most absorbent incontinence products.

Some toileting-program patients will stay dry on the 3-hour rounds, and with these patients it is possible to assess the efficiency of a 4-hour checking schedule. The same assessment procedure should be used during a second week to evaluate patients for a 4-hour schedule. The only difference is that the patient should be checked and toileted at 9:00 P.M., 1:00 A.M., and 5:00 A.M. Once again, if no skin irritation or wetness is noted during the 4-hour checks, the 4-hour schedule is justified.

QUALITY CONTROL OF NIGHTTIME PROGRAM

Quality control and management of the nighttime program utilize incontinence volumes as the primary quality-control measure. The pad-weighing and monitoring procedure used to control the quality of the daytime check–change program is also used at night. The same quality-assessment form (Chapter 6, Figure 6.6) can be used. The major difference is that the average 3-hour urine volumes of patients are used to set the expected 3-hour wetness levels and control limits. The expected levels of patient wetness are set during the 1-week assessment period. The average incontinent urine output of patients when they are checked on a 3-hour nighttime schedule is calculated in the same way as for the 2-hour volumes collected during the day. Once the average output is calculated by summarizing all 3-hour volumes and dividing by the total number of wet checks, either the standard deviation or the highest urine output over the 3-hour periods is calculated. If the standard deviation is used, the warning limit that signifies unusual patient wetness is set at two standard deviations above the average. If the highest volume is used, that number is the warning limit.

It is a good strategy to do one control check per night on each patient during the first month of the program. In addition, skin checks by a daytime nurse should be completed weekly on each patient for this first month. If no problems occur during this period (no out-of-control checks or skin irritation evidence), the control checks should be reduced to the same schedule utilized during the day. Thus, control checks two or three times per week should be adequate to maintain the program.

REFERENCES

Ancoli-Israel, S., Parker, L., Sinaee, R., Fell, R. L., & Kripke, D. F. (1989). Sleep fragmentation in patients from a nursing home. *Journal of Gerontology, 44*(1), 18–21.

Goldstein, L. A., & Goldstein, J. (1982). The Norton score: An early warning of pressure sores? *Journal of Advanced Nursing 7*, 419–426.

O'Donnell, P. D., Beck, C., & Walls, R. C. (1990). Serial incontinence assessment in elderly inpatient men. *Journal of Rehabilitation Research and Development, 27*(1), 1–8.

Sowell, V. A, Schnelle, J. F., Hu, T. W., & Traughber, B. (1987). A cost comparison of five methods of managing urinary incontinence. *Quality Review Bulletin, 13*, 411–414.

Taylor, K. J. (1988). Assessment tools for the identification of patients at risk for the development of pressure sores: A review. *Journal of Enterstomal Therapy, 15*(5), 201–205.

Chapter 8

INCONTINENCE MANAGEMENT AT HOME

What to learn from this chapter:

1. **How to assess incontinence problems for elderly people who can independently toilet.**
2. **How to measure independent toileting ability.**
3. **What types of incontinence-management procedures are used.**
4. **How to start an incontinence-management program for patients who live at home.**

Preceding chapters have emphasized treatment (Chapter 3), assessment (Chapter 4), and staff management procedures (Chapters 5, 6, and 7) that are most applicable to treating the physically dependent patient. Since most incontinent patients in nursing homes are dependent, these chapters are particularly important for nursing home care providers. Chapters 3 through 7 also emphasize nursing staff training and management because nursing staff play a critical role, not only in training patients to be continent but also in maintaining continence.

It is important to understand this distinction between training and maintenance. Training patients primarily refers to strengthening behaviors patients have already learned. For example, most patients already know how to toilet and how to respond to prompts for toileting assistance. The training program simply increases the frequency with which these learned behaviors are performed.

The maintenance of continence and toileting habits is a more vital issue in nursing home settings because most nursing home patients are so impaired that they will never be able to toilet independently. Thus, if continence is to be maintained, patients will always be dependent on staff for prompts, social reinforcement, and toileting assistance. If incontinent elderly patients living outside the nursing home are incapable of independent toileting, all of the procedures described in Chapters 3–7 are applicable. The only difference is that staff management and training procedures will have to be implemented by the home-care providers.

There are a small minority of nursing home patients and a larger majority of home-living elderly who are more capable of independent toileting. These latter patients are more physically and mentally intact than the typical nursing home patient. This chapter describes incontinence-management procedures that are relevant to these more independent patients. The first step in identifying these patients and understanding what to do with them is to assess independent toileting skills.

INDEPENDENCE VERSUS DEPENDENCE

There are three steps in assessing a patient's ability to toilet independently. The first step is a behavior rating scale that should be used by someone who knows the patient. This scale is an efficient way to assess whether a patient is physically capable of toileting independently with either a toilet, a bedpan, or a urinal. If a patient is rated as physically capable of independent toileting, the next step is a very brief behavioral screen of the patient's cognitive ability to use independent toileting skills. Some patients are physically capable of independent toileting but are so cognitively impaired that they remain dependent. The last step in the assessment process is a direct behavioral test of the patient's ability to toilet. This last test is a timed test that will provide useful information in determining what type of incontinence-management program should be used with the physically independent patient.

BEHAVIORAL RATING

It is not absolutely necessary that a patient be ambulatory to be independent. It is possible, although more difficult, for a nonambulatory patient to maintain toileting independence through the use of bedpans and urinals.

The physical skills needed to toilet independently are listed in Figure 8.1. Patients who are ambulatory with a cane or walker must be able to complete the first seven skills listed in the figure. Ambulatory patients who are rated "yes" on all seven skills are potentially capable of maintaining continence through independent use of a commode. Patients who are not ambulatory and who hope to maintain continence by use of a commode must be capable of the physical skills listed in items 8–14. Finally, nonambulatory patients who cannot do the transfer behaviors required in items 8–14 must have the skills listed in items 15–21.

Unfortunately, 88% of incontinent nursing home patients are not capable of independence with either a toilet, a bedpan, or a urinal. Incontinent patients are typically not ambulatory and do not have the transfer skills and strength needed to place themselves on and off toilet receptacles. Even if incontinent patients do have these basic physical skills (rated "yes" on items 1–7, 8–14, or 15–21), they may have severe cognitive problems that preclude independence.

COGNITIVE SCREEN

The next step in the assessment process is to determine if a patient has the necessary cognitive skills to maintain continence independently. Cognitive deficits that may preclude independent toileting are most noticeable in patients with severe dementias. For example, those with Alzheimer's disease typically show a profile of high levels of physical ability but very low levels of cognitive functioning. Alzheimer's disease patients may have a level of cognitive functioning so low that they cannot utilize their physical ability to maintain independence.

A good cognitive screen is to ask patients to show you the bathroom. If they cannot show you, their cognitive impairment precludes independent toileting. Such patients will be dependent on prompts from staff to maintain continence, and they should be managed with the prompted-voiding and assessment procedures

Name of Patient: ____________________
Name of Rater: ____________________
Date of Assessment: ____________________
This patient is: ____________________

Patient screening criteria:

A. If patient is ambulatory independently or with a cane/walker, complete items 1–21.
B. If patient spends a majority of waking hours in a wheelchair, complete items 8–21.
C. If the patient spends a majority of waking hours in bed, complete items 15–21.

Please circle yes or No in response to the following questions based on your observations. Please make your determinations on the basis of what the patient actually does rather that what you feel he or she might be capable of doing.

1. Does patient get up from chair independently? yes or no
2. Does patient get up from bed independently? yes or no
3. Does patient walk without staff assistance to commode from any point in the room? yes or no
4. Does patient sit on commode independently? yes or no
5. Does patient rise from commode independently? yes or no
6. Does patient remove clothing independently? yes or no
7. Does patient clean self independently? yes or no
8. Does patient assist in transfer from bed to wheelchair? yes or no
9. Does patient bear partial weight and assist in transfer from chair to wheelchair? yes or no
10. Does patient wheel self to commode or bathroom independently? yes or no
11. Does patient bear partial weight and assist in transfer from chair to commode? yes or no
12. Does patient bear partial weight and assist in transfer from commode to wheelchair? yes or no
13. Does patient clean self independently? yes or no
14. Does patient remove clothing independently? yes or no
15. Does patient grasp urinal or bedpan from bed position? yes or no
16. Does patient grasp urinal or bedpan from chair position? yes or no
17. Does patient place bedpan or urinal in position from chair? yes or no
18. Does patient place bedpan or urinal in position from bed? yes or no
19. Does patient successfully remove clothes from either chair or bed? yes or no
20. Does patient remove bedpan or urinal successfully after using? yes or no
21. Does patient clean self successfully from either bed or chair position? yes or no

FIGURE 8.1 Independent toileting assessment inventory.

described in Chapters 3–7. If physically capable patients pass the simple cognitive screen, their ability to toilet can be assessed more precisely with a timed independent-toileting assessment test called the "potti." This test evaluates a patient's ability to do most of the critical cognitive and physical skills needed to toilet independently.

POTTI TEST

The potti test, described by Ouslander, Morishita, Blaustein, Orzeck, Dunn, and Sayre (1987), can be used with patients who are rated as physically and cognitively capable of independent toileting (passed assessment steps 1 and 2). In this test patients are asked to perform a series of timed manual tasks related to toileting. The tasks include moving 15 feet to the toilet, transferring to a commode, unfastening a hook, unzipping a zipper, and pulling off an apron or gown.

First place the patient in a sitting position 15 feet from the toilet with an apron-like garment on. The apron should have a zipper and a hook. Second, instruct the patient to walk to the bathroom. The amount of time it takes to walk to the bathroom is timed to a maximum of 55 seconds. Patients who cannot or will not move to the toilet should be given a maximum time of 55 seconds. Once in the proximity of the toilet, ask the patient to sit. This task is also timed, up to a maximum of 55 seconds. Inability or refusal to perform this task is once again given the maximum time. Once sitting, the patient should be instructed to unhook the hook, timed for a maximum of 35 seconds. Next ask the patient to unzip the zipper (maximum time, 25 seconds) and to remove the garment (maximum time, 25 seconds). Patients who score low times on the potti test are most capable of independent toileting. The average continent patient can complete all of the tasks in 60 seconds.

If patients complete all of the tasks but do so very slowly (over 100 seconds), they may have difficulties maintaining continence independently. These slow patients should probably be managed with the same prompted-voiding procedures that are used with the more physically dependent patients. Similarly, patients who fail on any one of the potti tasks because of inability to comprehend instructions or because of physical problems probably could best be managed with the prompted-voiding procedures. In either of the latter cases (unusually slow times on all tasks or failure on one task) the patient will be dependent on a caregiver for toileting assistance.

Patients who complete all toileting tasks in a reasonable amount of time (approximately 60 to 100 seconds) probably have the physical and mental skills necessary to toilet independently. Efforts to control incontinence through one of the management procedures for patients who can toilet independently can now be attempted. These techniques are described in this chapter.

INCONTINENCE IN INDEPENDENT ELDERLY

Recent surveys by Diokno, Brock, Brown, and Herzog (1988) suggest that about 30% of all independent-living elderly patients suffer some involuntary urine loss. Nearly twice as many women (37.7%) as men (18.9%) are affected by this problem. Although the amounts and frequency of urine loss may vary, the majority report moderate amounts (greater than one half teaspoon of urine per episode) occurring more than 10 days per year. Approximately 30% of those reporting incontinent symptoms voided more than nine times per day. Most were more likely to be incontinent during the day than during the night.

Urge symptoms are the most frequently reported symptoms among men, whereas women report a mixture of urge and stress symptoms. As discussed in Chapter 1, urge incontinence results because the interval between the sensation to void and the actual voiding does not allow time to reach a toileting receptacle. Stress incontinence—leakage of urine produced by coughing, laughing, or other stressful movements—is often mixed with the inability to reach the bathroom in time.

In addition to the more prevalent stress, urge, or mixed incontinence, a significant number (18% men and 9% women) report difficulties with bladder emptying. Among men prostatic enlargement with outlet obstruction is the most common cause for incomplete bladder emptying. Women, on the other hand, often develop emptying difficulties when the bladder looses elasticity. A history of infrequent voiding patterns may result in chronic overdistention of the bladder. This in turn leads to loss of elasticity and inability to empty the bladder.

Because current studies have not been conducted among independent elderly living in nursing homes, no one knows the actual occurrence of incontinence among patients classified by staff as continent. It is known, however, that the majority (91%) of those rated as continent are capable of independent toileting (Schnelle, Sowell, Traughber, & Hu 1988). This independent capability is the primary factor that allows the nursing home patient to remain continent. It would not be surprising, however, to discover that some of these "continent" patients show occasional episodes of urine loss similar to their independent counterparts in the community. Perhaps the nursing home staff is unaware of incontinent episodes among these "continent" patients who can independently toilet and change their own soiled clothing. Perhaps the amount of urine loss is far less severe among these independent nursing home patients than among the more dependent patients. In any case, efforts to document the presence of incontinence among independent nursing home residents should be initiated.

Regardless of residence (i.e., home vs. nursing home environment), any independent elderly person affected by occasional incontinent episodes can receive the same assessment and management procedures.

MANAGEMENT OF URINARY INCONTINENCE

Chapter 1 distinguishes between management and treatment approaches to incontinence problems. The management approach is defined as efforts by caregivers and patients to compensate for problems that make incontinence more likely or more frequent. In the case of the physically or cognitively dependent patient, the management approach emphasizes efforts to provide more frequent toileting assistance and to keep patients' attention on their incontinence status. Thus, the systematic prompted-voiding procedure helps compensate for physical and cognitive dependence and even some of the urological problems that make incontinence severe in the dependent nursing home patient. The primary advantages of the management approach is that it remains noninvasive and relatively inexpensive and can be attempted by a trained nurse, caregiver, or patient.

The treatment approach is directed more toward the cause of the incontinence. Thus, surgical procedures and medications designed to improve bladder functioning would be examples of the treatment approach, as would biofeedback procedures that involve either catheterization or instrumentation to implement the therapy.

The treatment approach requires professional assistance and is more invasive and expensive than the management approach. Despite these disadvantages, medical consultation for urinary incontinence problems is clearly advisable for all incontinent patients. Patients capable of independent toileting are less frail than more dependent patients and are probably better candidates for invasive medical or behavioral treatments. In addition, a medical evaluation may reveal factors contributing to incontinence that can be easily reversed. Thus, medical evaluation and treatment could increase the probability that the management procedures will work.

This chapter advises medical consultation but continues to emphasize the management approach even for those patients capable of independent toileting. The management approach can be attempted without significant risk and, at the very least, serves as a useful supplement to medical treatment. In some cases the management approach will solve the incontinence problem.

To introduce management strategies, it is helpful to describe what types of incontinence management people normally attempt. Surveys have been conducted with 2,000 incontinent people who were asked to describe the types of things they do to control their incontinence (Herzog, Fultz, Normolle, Brock, & Diokno, 1989). These surveys indicate that the most popular control method is use of absorbent materials. Finding a toilet upon arrival at a location and scheduling or increasing voiding attempts are the next two most popular procedures.

Absorbent products (briefs, pads, diapers) are often effective in containing urine and in controlling the visible signs of incontinence. Many patients report more confidence and a feeling of freedom to go to public places when using absorbent briefs. Obviously, absorbent materials contain urine loss, but they do so without reducing the frequency or severity of urine loss. The primary danger of absorbent products is that people will use them exclusively and not try other potentially beneficial procedures.

The ideal situation would be to use absorbent products to increase comfort or confidence but at the same time try other management procedures described in this chapter. In general, absorbent products should not be used as the only incontinence-management strategy unless all other strategies have failed. Absorbent products remain a very useful and important management strategy, either as a supplement to other procedures or as the primary management strategy if other strategies do not work.

The strategy of locating a toilet upon arrival and increasing the frequency of voiding illustrates the single most useful component of all incontinence-management strategies. It is not surprising that many people have discovered the value of these procedures on their own.

Locating a toilet reduces the amount of time a patient needs to find a toilet when feeling the urge to void. In cases where there is a small delay between sensation and actual voiding, the time saved by knowing a toilet's location can be critical.

Increasing the frequency of voiding or scheduling times for voiding episodes can be effective with both stress and urge incontinence. Increasing voiding frequency obviously means less urine in the bladder. Thus, the bladder is not stretched to the point that there is a high pressure or a need to void. Stressful events, such as coughs, are less likely to cause leakage in bladders that are not filled. In addition, a less full bladder will probably invite fewer episodes in which urge symptoms are felt.

A major problem with the frequent-voiding toileting strategy is that it can become cumbersome and limiting to some patients. For example, having to void every hour to feel comfortable and to control urine loss is time-consuming and restrictive. A bladder drill strategy designed to increase intervals between required voidings is advisable in such cases.

In summary, many elderly people have invented or naturally come to utilize incontinence management strategies, which are used because they work. The remainder of this chapter describes how these management strategies can best be planned, implemented, and evaluated for patients capable of independent toileting.

TIMED VOIDING MANAGEMENT

Timed voiding management is probably most useful for patients who feel minimal sensation prior to voiding and for people who have difficulty emptying the bladder. In this approach a fixed voiding schedule is set, and the patient attempts to void at designated hours. The actual voiding schedule is usually set for every 2 hours during the day and less frequently during the night. The logic of timed voiding is obviously to keep bladder pressure at a relatively low level so as to reduce the probability of an accident. If people receive little notice or sensation of bladder pressure, such a simple approach is compelling. If the 2-hour schedule works in reducing incontinence episodes, it should be possible to attempt a 3-hour schedule. If the 2-hour schedule does not work, reducing the schedule to 1 or 1.5 hours is simply too restrictive for most people. Other management techniques should be tried if the 2-hour schedule fails.

There are several types of exercises or strategies people can use during the timed voiding attempts to promote better bladder emptying or to start the voiding process. If people on a 2-hour schedule have difficulty starting the voiding process or void small amounts (less than 100 cc), an effort could be made to empty the bladder more completely. For example, techniques such as running water or stroking the inner thigh may enhance the voiding process. In addition, straining exercises such as bending forward and pushing on the lower abdomen may improve emptying (Kane, Ouslander, & Abrass, 1989; Resnick, Yalla, & Laurino, 1989).

BLADDER TRAINING

The bladder training or bladder drill approach, unlike timed voiding, is designed to gradually increase patients' bladder capacity and ability to hold urine. Bladder training is most useful for patients with urge symptoms who still have some sensation of bladder pressure prior to voiding.

The patient begins the program exactly like a timed-voiding program in that attempts to use the bathroom are made every 2 hours. If successful at maintaining continence on a 2-hour schedule, the patient extends the voiding intervals to a maximum of 3 or 4 hours. If incontinence persists on a 2-hour schedule, the voiding intervals are reduced until continence is achieved. Intervals can then be gradually lengthened again.

Patients are sometimes instructed not to use the toilet between scheduled voiding intervals even at the cost of becoming incontinent. Other programs instruct patients to try to hold their urine, but if the urge becomes unbearable, they may use the toilet. Most independent and cognitively intact patients who attempt this procedure can probably utilize the wait-but-go-if-necessary strategy. Such a strategy requires more judgment and discipline on the part of the patient, but it is judgment that the successful patient should have.

The most difficult aspect of bladder drill is to change the voiding intervals progressively on a timely basis. It is vital that voiding intervals be changed as patients improve incontinence rates. Records of both volume and episodes of continence thus become vital. The chart shown in Figure 8.2 is useful in this scheduling program.

The patient should be started on a 2-hour schedule and instructed as follows:

> We will start the program at 8:00 A.M., and you should try to use the bathroom at 8:00 A.M., 10:00 A.M., noon, 2:00 P.M., 4:00 P.M., 6:00 P.M., and 8:00 P.M. It is important that you try really hard not to use the bathroom between the scheduled voiding times. So try to use the bathroom at 8:00 A.M., but don't use it again until 10:00 A.M. If you absolutely can't stop yourself from going between 8:00 and 10:00 you can use the bathroom. Mark an X in the urge column when you feel a desire to void. Once again, remember, try to control the urge and don't use the bathroom between the

	Urge to Void	Accident (record "large" or "small")	Toilet (record voided volume)
8:00			
8:30			
9:00			
9:30			
10:30			
11:00			
11:30			
12:00			
12:30			
1:00			
1:30			
2:00			
2:30			
3:00			
3:30			
4:00			
4:30			
5:00			
5:30			
6:00			
6:30			
7:00			
7:30			
8:00			
8:30			
9:00			
9:30			
10:00			

FIGURE 8.2 Bladder drill schedule.

> 2-hour scheduled voiding times. Void only at the 2-hour intervals and record all accidents or toiletings that occur on the 2-hour chart [see Figure 8.2]. Write the volume of the void in the "Toilet" column every time you use the toilet. Write "0" if you try to use the toilet and don't produce a measurable void. Each time you use the toilet, you should measure the volume of the void with a toilet insert. Write "large" or "small" in the "Accident" column when you have an accident.

If there is less than one small wet episode per day for 10 days on the 2-hour schedule, the patient can be moved to a 2.5-hour schedule. All instructions and charting rules continue to apply for the 2.5-hour schedule. The only difference is that the patient toilets at 8:00 A.M., 10:30 A.M., 1:00 P.M., 3:30 P.M., 6:00 P.M., and 8:30 P.M. If the 2.5-hour schedule is successful for 10 days (less than one small wet episode per day), efforts can be made to use a 3-hour schedule, a 3.5-hour schedule, and finally a 4-hour schedule. The same rules apply to each schedule, and each should be attempted for 10 days before a decision is made about its success. If a patient continues to have more than one accident per day on a 2-hour schedule, a 1.5-hour schedule can be attempted and then gradually extended back up the range of hours.

It is sometimes useful to graph patients' average urinary output per toileting for each day they are on the bladder drill program. Toileting inserts are used to capture and measure the volume of voids in a toilet. The patient simply adds all of the voids in the toilet that occurred during the day and divides by the number of toileting times.

These average daily outputs can be graphed on a chart such as that shown in Figure 8.3. Optimally, urine output will show a gradual increase over time, reflecting larger voluntary voids, few-

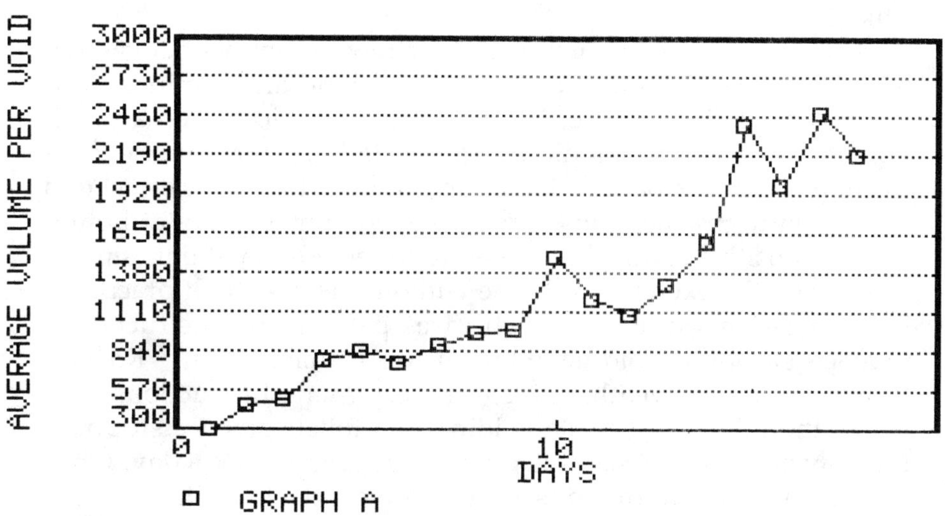

FIGURE 8.3 Graph of average daily urinary output.

er accidents, and a larger bladder capacity. This ideal scenario is illustrated with hypothetical data graphed on Figure 8.3.

The graphing step is optional and should not be attempted if patients or other caregivers do not understand how to graph or how to calculate an average. The advantage of graphing is that it can serve as a motivating stimulus to the patient in the same way that charting weight loss motivates a patient on a diet. The graph serves as a visible sign of progress that motivates people to maintain the toileting regimen.

MUSCLE RETRAINING STRATEGY

Muscle retraining to manage stress incontinence was first described by Kegel (1948). The logic of the Kegel exercises is to reduce stress leakage by increasing the strength and efficiency of pelvic-floor muscles. Contracting these muscles should counteract the pressure to void that is produced by coughs and other stressful stimuli that increase bladder pressure and cause stress leakage.

Most typically, the patient is taught how to contract her vaginal muscles by contracting these muscles around an examiner's finger in a physician's office. In some cases a device called a pereinometer is used to monitor the strength of the muscle contractions. Once a patient learns to contract the muscles, she is instructed to practice the exercises several times a day at home.

Some positive results have been reported when patients simply learn to do the exercises at home without the benefit of practicing in a physician's office. In such cases patients are instructed to practice stopping voiding while using a toilet. Mohr, Rogers, Brown, and Starkweather (1983), report giving instructions similar to the following: While voiding in a toilet, practice stopping the flow of urine. Repeat this procedure several times a day. Once you are sensitive to the muscles you are contracting that stop the flow, practice contracting these muscles two or three times per day for 10 minutes while not voiding. Repeat these exercises for at least 10 days.

The outcome of practicing the Kegel exercises without specific training in the physician's office or the use of a pereinometer have been mixed. However, since some reports have been positive and since the procedures are so simple, it is probably worthwhile to try these exercises at home for 10 or 15 days. Since many women show both urge and stress incontinence symptoms, these simple muscle exercises can be attempted at the same time as the bladder drill or timed voiding strategies.

In addition to the management strategies described in this book, there are numerous other treatment alternatives available. Alternative medical and behavioral treatments have proved effective in treating many types of incontinence, but they require some professional consultation to implement. A good urologist or geriatric nurse practitioner should be able to provide information to patients about alternative treatments.

The management strategies described in this book do work, but their efficiency and simplicity should not prevent the patient or caregiver from seeking professional consultation. Most professionals will probably advise the use of management strategies either in conjunction with or instead of the more invasive medical treatments.

Knowledge of how to manage incontinence is an important first step in addressing the problem. It is the responsibility of all people who care for the elderly to have this knowledge. All informed patients and caregivers should be capable of implementing the simple assessment and management strategies described in this book. There is an excellent chance that systematic application of this management technology will produce noticeable improvement in incontinence problems.

REFERENCES

Diokno, A. C., Brock, B. M., Brown, M. B., & Herzog, A. R. (1986). Prevalence of urinary incontinence and other urological symptoms in the noninstitutionalized elderly. *The Journal of Urology, 13,* 1022–1025.

Herzog, A. R., Fultz, N. H., Normolle, D. P., Brock, B. M., & Diokno, A. C. (1989). Methods used to manage urinary incontinence by older adults in the community. *Journal of American Geriatric Society, 37,* 339–347.

Kane, R., Ouslander, J. G., & Abrass, I. (1989). *Essentials of clinical geriatrics* (2nd ed.). New York: McGraw-Hill.

Kegel, A. H. (1948). Progressive resistance exercise in the functional restoration of the perineal muscles. *American Journal of Obstetrics and Gynecology, 56,* 238–248.

Mohr, J. A., Rogers, J., Jr., Brown, T. N., & Starkweather, G. (1983). Stress urinary incontinence: A simple and practical approach to diagnosis and treatment. *Journal of American Geriatric Society, 31,* 476–478.

Ouslander, J. G., Morishita, L., Blaustein, J., Orzeck, S., Dunn, S., & Sayre, J. (1987). Clinical, functional, and psychosocial characteristics of an incontinent nursing home population. *Journal of Gerontology, 42*(6), 631–637.

Resnick, N., Yalla, S., & Laurino, E. (1989). The pathophysiology of urinary incontinence among institutionalized elderly persons. *New England Journal of Medicine, 320*(1), 1–7.

Schnelle, J. F., Sowell, V. A., Traughber, G., & Hu, T. W. (1988). A behavioral analysis of the labor cost of managing continence and incontinence in nursing home patients. *Journal of Organizational Behavior Management, 9*(2), 137–153.

APPENDIX A

LETTER OF EXPLANATION

Dear ______:

We are happy to have ______ as a new resident. We will make every effort to offer the most professional and caring nursing service that can be provided. One part of our effort will be to assess the incontinence problems of ______. We are required to both assess and treat the incontinence problems of each individual patient. The assessment process involves checking a patient every two hours and offering toileting assistance. We also measure the size or volume of the patients' voids for six days.

Based on this information we will attempt to manage the patients' continence either by offering toileting assistance every two hours or by changing the patient every two hours. Patients will be offered toileting assistance every two hours only if the assessment information indicates that such toileting assistance will be beneficial.

The goal of all our efforts is to keep the patient as dry and comfortable as possible. We can assure you that our efforts are based on the most recent knowledge in the field and that the nursing residents are receiving the best professional nursing care that is possible.

If we can answer questions about out program, do not hesitate to call any of the staff members listed at the bottom of this letter. We look forward to taking care of Mrs. ______.

Sincerely,

APPENDIX **B**

CHECKLIST FOR ASSESSMENT DAYS 1–6

Items needed for each patient:

Weighed blue pads

Weighed diapers

Peel-off labels

Inserts/bedpans

Baby wipes
(1 box per patient)

Small trash bags

Other general items needed:

Assessment sheet for apropriate assessment day

Large trash bags for disposal of wet pads/diapers

Scale

Calculator

15 extra weighed pads

10 extra weighed diapers

Box of extra pens

ASSESSMENT SHEET FOR TOILETING PROGRAM: DAY 1

Patient Name ____________
Nurse's Name ____________
Date ____________

Checks	Wetness		Toileting		Responsiveness			Volume	
No. of checks made	Patient was (Circle one)		Did patient use the toilet? Yes: Urine or BM No: No attempt		Did patient answer question of wet or dry? (Circle One)			CC of void	
7:00 A.M.	wet	dry	yes	no	yes correct	yes incorrect	no answer	cont. ____	incont. ____
9:00 A.M.	wet	dry	yes	no	yes correct	yes incorrect	no answer	cont. ____	incont. ____
11:00 A.M.	wet	dry	yes	no	yes correct	yes incorrect	no answer	cont. ____	incont. ____
1:00 P.M.	wet	dry	yes	no	yes correct	yes incorrect	no answer	cont. ____	incont. ____
3:00 P.M.	wet	dry	yes	no	yes correct	yes incorrect	no answer	cont. ____	incont. ____
5:00 P.M.	wet	dry	yes	no	yes correct	yes incorrect	no answer	cont. ____	incont. ____
7:00 P.M.	wet	dry	yes	no	yes correct	yes incorrect	no answer	cont. ____	incont. ____

Summary	Total number of wets	Total number of toilets	Total # correct	Total # incorrect	Total # no answer	Total cont. cc	Total incont. cc
9:00 A.M. to 7:00 P.M.	____	____	____	____	____	____	____

[____ / (____ + ____)] = ____ % Appropriate toileting

Decision Point:

If there are any "Yes" responses in either Toileting or Responsiveness columns, continue patient on prompted voiding for the second day. If there are no "Yes" responses, put patient on check-change protocol. Calculate % Appropriate Toilets by dividing Total # of Toilets by Total # of wets + Total # of Toilets.

ASSESSMENT SHEET FOR TOILETING PROGRAM: DAY 2

Patient Name ____________
Nurse's Name ____________
Date ____________

Checks	Wetness		Toileting		Responsiveness			Volume	
No. of checks made	Patient was (Circle one)		Did patient use the toilet? Yes: Urine or BM No: No attempt		Did patient answer question of wet or dry? (Circle One)			CC of void	
7:00 A.M.	wet	dry	yes	no	yes correct	yes incorrect	no answer	cont.	incont
9:00 A.M.	wet	dry	yes	no	yes correct	yes incorrect	no answer	cont.	incont
11:00 A.M.	wet	dry	yes	no	yes correct	yes incorrect	no answer	cont.	incont
1:00 P.M.	wet	dry	yes	no	yes correct	yes incorrect	no answer	cont.	incont
3:00 P.M.	wet	dry	yes	no	yes correct	yes incorrect	no answer	cont.	incont
5:00 P.M.	wet	dry	yes	no	yes correct	yes incorrect	no answer	cont.	incont
7:00 P.M.	wet	dry	yes	no	yes correct	yes incorrect	no answer	cont.	incont

Summary	Total number of wets	Total number of toilets	Total # correct	Total # incorrect	Total # no answer	Total cont. cc	Total incont cc
9:00 A.M. to 7:00 P.M.	____	____	____	____	____	____	____

____________ (over) ____ + ____ = ____ % Appropriate toileting

Decision Point:

There must be a "Yes" response in both Toileting or Responsiveness columns. If so, continue patient on prompted voiding for the third day. If there is not a "Yes" response in both columns put patient on check-change protocol.

ASSESSMENT SHEET FOR TOILETING PROGRAM: DAY 3

Patient Name ____________
Nurse's Name ____________
Date ____________

Checks	Wetness		Toileting		Responsiveness			Volume	
No. of checks made	Patient was (Circle one)		Did patient use the toilet? Yes: Urine or BM No: No attempt		Did patient answer question of wet or dry? (Circle One)			CC of void	
7:00 A.M.	wet	dry	yes	no	yes correct	yes incorrect	no answer	cont.	incont.
9:00 A.M.	wet	dry	yes	no	yes correct	yes incorrect	no answer	cont.	incont.
11:00 A.M.	wet	dry	yes	no	yes correct	yes incorrect	no answer	cont.	incont.
1:00 P.M.	wet	dry	yes	no	yes correct	yes incorrect	no answer	cont.	incont.
3:00 P.M.	wet	dry	yes	no	yes correct	yes incorrect	no answer	cont.	incont.
5:00 P.M.	wet	dry	yes	no	yes correct	yes incorrect	no answer	cont.	incont.
7:00 P.M.	wet	dry	yes	no	yes correct	yes incorrect	no answer	cont.	incont.

Summary	Total number of wets	Total number of toilets	Total # correct	Total # incorrect	Total # no answer	Total cont. cc	Total incont. cc
9:00 A.M. to 7:00 P.M.	____	____	____	____	____	____	____

________ (total number of toilets)
____ + ____ (total number of wets + total number of toilets)
= ____ % Appropriate toileting

Decision Point:

No decisions: continue prompted voiding patients on prompted void protocol. Continue check-change patients on check-change protocol.

ASSESSMENT SHEET FOR TOILETING PROGRAM: DAY 4

Patient Name ____________
Nurse's Name ____________
Date ____________

Checks	Wetness		Toileting		Responsiveness			Volume	
No. of checks made	Patient was (Circle one)		Did patient use the toilet? Yes: Urine or BM No: No attempt		Did patient answer question of wet or dry? (Circle One)			CC of void	
7:00 A.M.	wet	dry	yes	no	yes correct	yes incorrect	no answer	cont. ___	incont. ___
9:00 A.M.	wet	dry	yes	no	yes correct	yes incorrect	no answer	cont. ___	incont. ___
11:00 A.M.	wet	dry	yes	no	yes correct	yes incorrect	no answer	cont. ___	incont. ___
1:00 P.M.	wet	dry	yes	no	yes correct	yes incorrect	no answer	cont. ___	incont. ___
3:00 P.M.	wet	dry	yes	no	yes correct	yes incorrect	no answer	cont. ___	incont. ___
5:00 P.M.	wet	dry	yes	no	yes correct	yes incorrect	no answer	cont. ___	incont. ___
7:00 P.M.	wet	dry	yes	no	yes correct	yes incorrect	no answer	cont. ___	incont. ___

Summary	Total number of wets	Total number of toilets	Total # correct	Total # incorrect	Total # no answer	Total cont. cc	Total incont. cc
9:00 A.M. to 7:00 P.M.	___	___	___	___	___	___	___

______ ÷ (___ + ___) = ___ % Appropriate toileting

Decision Point:

Patient must show an appropriate toilet percentage of 50% to continue in Prompted Voiding. Below 50% toileting should go to check-change protocol.

ASSESSMENT SHEET FOR TOILETING PROGRAM: DAY 5

Patient Name ____________
Nurse's Name ____________
Date ____________

Checks	Wetness		Toileting		Responsiveness			Volume	
No. of checks made	Patient was (Circle one)		Did patient use the toilet? Yes: Urine or BM No: No attempt		Did patient answer question of wet or dry? (Circle One)			CC of void	
7:00 A.M.	wet	dry	yes	no	yes correct	yes incorrect	no answer	cont. ____	incont. ____
9:00 A.M.	wet	dry	yes	no	yes correct	yes incorrect	no answer	cont. ____	incont. ____
11:00 A.M.	wet	dry	yes	no	yes correct	yes incorrect	no answer	cont. ____	incont. ____
1:00 P.M.	wet	dry	yes	no	yes correct	yes incorrect	no answer	cont. ____	incont. ____
3:00 P.M.	wet	dry	yes	no	yes correct	yes incorrect	no answer	cont. ____	incont. ____
5:00 P.M.	wet	dry	yes	no	yes correct	yes incorrect	no answer	cont. ____	incont. ____
7:00 P.M.	wet	dry	yes	no	yes correct	yes incorrect	no answer	cont. ____	incont. ____

Summary	Total number of wets	Total number of toilets	Total # correct	Total # incorrect	Total # no answer	Total cont. cc	Total incont. cc
9:00 A.M. to 7:00 P.M.	____	____	____	____	____	____	____

$$\frac{\text{\_\_\_\_\_\_ (total number of toilets)}}{\text{\_\_\_ (total number of wets)} + \text{\_\_\_ (total number of toilets)}} = \text{\_\_\_}$$ % Appropriate toileting

Decision Point:

No decision: continue prompted voiding patients in prompted voiding and check-change patient in check-change protocol.

ASSESSMENT SHEET FOR TOILETING PROGRAM: DAY 6

Patient Name ____________
Nurse's Name ____________
Date ____________

Checks	Wetness		Toileting		Responsiveness			Volume	
No. of checks made	Patient was (Circle one)		Did patient use the toilet? Yes: Urine or BM No: No attempt		Did patient answer question of wet or dry? (Circle One)			CC of void	
7:00 A.M.	wet	dry	yes	no	yes correct	yes incorrect	no answer	cont. ____	incont. ____
9:00 A.M.	wet	dry	yes	no	yes correct	yes incorrect	no answer	cont. ____	incont. ____
11:00 A.M.	wet	dry	yes	no	yes correct	yes incorrect	no answer	cont. ____	incont. ____
1:00 P.M.	wet	dry	yes	no	yes correct	yes incorrect	no answer	cont. ____	incont. ____
3:00 P.M.	wet	dry	yes	no	yes correct	yes incorrect	no answer	cont. ____	incont. ____
5:00 P.M.	wet	dry	yes	no	yes correct	yes incorrect	no answer	cont. ____	incont. ____
7:00 P.M.	wet	dry	yes	no	yes correct	yes incorrect	no answer	cont. ____	incont. ____

Summary	Total number of wets	Total number of toilets	Total # correct	Total # incorrect	Total # no answer	Total cont. cc	Total incont. cc
9:00 A.M. to 7:00 P.M.	____	____	____	____	____	____	____

____________ ← = ____ % Appropriate toileting

→ ____ + ____ ←

Decision Point:
Summarize all data on final assessment summary sheet.

FINAL ASSESSMENT SUMMARY SHEET AND TREATMENT DECISION

Patient's Name ____________
Date ____________

Toileting Ability

Appropriate Toileting %	Check Appr. Box
0%–65% Poor ability to toilet	______
66%–75% Average ability to toilet	______
75%–100% Excellent ability to toilet	______

Bladder Storage Ability

Frequency of wets per day:

0–1 Good ability to prevent incontinence	______
1–2 Marginal ability to prevent incontinence	______
2+ Poor ability to prevent incontinence	______

Volume of wets per day:

0–30 cc Good ability to control urine loss	______
30–75 cc Marginal ability to control urine loss	______
75+ cc Poor ability to control urine loss	______

Mental Responsiveness

No question answered—poor responsiveness	______
Answered 50% correctly—marginal responsiveness	______
Answered 75% correctly—excellent responsiveness	______

6-Day Assessment Summary

Toileting ability

Column
1 total no. wets
2 total no. toilets
3 total no. voids (columns 1 + 2)
4 % appr. toilet $\frac{\text{(column 2)}}{\text{(column 3)}}$

Storage ability

Responsiveness

Column
8 no. yes correct responses
9% correct $\frac{\text{(col. 8)}}{\text{no. days in prompted voiding} \times 6} =$

5 No. expected wets per day $\frac{\text{(total wets)}}{6}$ =

6 Avg. vol. inc. episodes
$\frac{\text{(add all inc. vols)}}{\text{(column 1)}}$ =

7 Lowest inc. vol ______
Largest Inc. vol ______

APPENDIX C

PROMPTED VOIDING CHECKLIST

Date: ______ Time: ______ Patient: ______
Person Observed: ______ Person Observing: ______

	Yes	No	Doesn't apply
1. Greet the patient by name?	____	____	______
2. Check urinal, bedpan, and commode to see if the patient has toileted without assistance since last check?	____	____	______
3. Praise the patient if s/he has toileted without assistance?	____	____	______
4. Ask patient "Do you feel wet or do you feel dry?"	____	____	______
5. Ask again if the patient does not answer?	____	____	______
6. Feel the patient's clothes, bedding, and body to see if the patient is wet or dry?	____	____	______
7. Tell patient whether or not s/he was correct or incorrect about being dry or wet?	____	____	______
8. Praise the patient if s/he was dry? ("You're doing a great job of staying dry today.")	____	____	______
9. Correct the patient if s/he was wet? ("From now on, let me know when you want to go to the bathroom. Don't wet on yourself.")	____	____	______
10. Praise the patient if s/he asks for toileting assistance?	____	____	______
11. Assist the patient to toilet if s/he asks for assistance?	____	____	______
12. Ask the patient if s/he will try to use the bathroom if the patient hasn't asked for assistance?	____	____	______

	Yes	No	Doesn't apply
13. Ask again if the patient does not say yes?	_____	_____	_______
14. Ask a third time if the patient does not say yes?	_____	_____	_______
15. Take patient to toilet only if the patient says s/he will try to use the bathroom?	_____	_____	_______
16. Praise the patient for trying to use the bathroom?	_____	_____	_______
17. Write toileting information on patient sheets?	_____	_____	_______
18. Wash hands?	_____	_____	_______
19. Pour water and offer to patient if in patient's room?	_____	_____	_______
20. Tell patient that someone will check back with him/her in about 2 hours?	_____	_____	_______

FLOOR SUPERVISOR JOB CHECKLIST AND RANDOM HOUR CHECKS

Prior to beginning report, be sure the clipboards are ready for aides to pick up at the beginning of shift.

Make sure clipboards are turned in during last 30 minutes of the shift. Discourage turning in boards earlier.

Conduct random checks on the incontinent states of patients and on toileting records. The checks should proceed as listed below:

If you find any of the following:

1. The clipboard is not in the patient's room.
2. The form is full and has not been replaced by a new form.
3. The patient's name is not written on the sheet.
4. The aide's name is not written on the sheet.
5. The date is not written on the sheet.

You should:

1. Within 30 minutes, notify the aide of the error, stressing that you want the error corrected within the next 30 minutes.
2. Verify that the problem has been corrected.
3. If the error has not been corrected, repeat 1 and 2.

If you find any of the following:

1. There is an empty 2-hour block.
2. There is an aide check in which the "void correctly" symbol is filled in, but there is no indication if the patient has been dry or incontinent.

You should:

1. Circle the error.
2. Write the words "aide error" next to the error.

If you find the patient wet, you should:

Write in "W," the time, and your initials immediately after you do the check.

If you find the patient dry, you should:

Write in "D," the time, and your initials immediately after you do the check.

JOB DESCRIPTION FOR NURSE'S AIDES

Once you have clocked in and picked up your assignments for the day, these things are to be done before anything else:

1. Immediately pick up the clipboards for the patients on the program that you have for the day. If the clipboard is not at the nurses' station, check the patient's room.

2. Make sure that the toileting record form is not full and you have space to fill in your information to be collected that day. If the sheet is full (front and back), immediately pick up a blank sheet from the notebook at the nurses' station and put the full sheet under the patient's name in the notebook.

3. Go immediately to the rooms of each of the patients you have for the day who are on the program.

4. Hang the board on the bathroom door, filling in your name, date, and patient's name if necessary.

5. Do the prompted-voiding procedure.

6. Repeat the prompted-voiding procedure every 2 hours throughout the day.

7. In the last hour of your shift turn your clipboards in at the nurses' station for the next shift. Clipboards should not be turned in until 15 minutes before shift is over.

8. You are expected to have information on the clipboard as to the patient's condition in the first and last hour of your shift and every 2 hours in between. This applies to all shifts.

9. Change the patients on the program immediately if they are found wet within any 2-hour round. Try to toilet these patients and not rely on frequent changes.

PROGRAM START-UP TASKS

6:45 A.M. Give aides and the floor supervisors the job behavior checklist, and take all aides on one prompted-voiding round.

11:00 A.M. Check the patient's chart and warn the floor nurses of any major problems.

2:45 P.M. Make sure the charts are returned to the nurses' station. Review the charts and note unusual recordings. Be particularly sure that floor nurses make at least one check on the patient during that shift.

3:00 P.M. Take new group of aides on training round.

6:00 P.M. Check patients' charts in the rooms and alert floor nurse to potential problems.

10:45 P.M. Make sure the charts are returned to the nurses' station. Review charts for errors or inaccurate recording. Give feedback to nurses concerning problems.

APPENDIX D

EXAMPLE OF CALCULATIONS

Patient	Assessment Days					
	1	2	3	4	5	6
1	DWDDDD	WDDDDW	DDDDDD	WWDDDD	DDDDDD	WDDWDD
2	DDDDDD	DWDDDD	WWDDDD	DDDDDD	WDDDDD	DDDDDD
3	WDDDDD	WWDDDD	DDDDDD	WDDDDD	DDDDDD	WDDDDD
4	DDDDDD	DDDDDD	WDDDDD	DDDDDD	WDDDDD	DDDDDD
5	WDDDDD	DDDDDD	WDDDDD	WDDDDD	DDDDDD	WDDDDD
6	DDDDDD	WDDDDD	DWWWDD	DDDDDD	DDDDDD	WDDDDD
7	DWWDDD	DDDDDD	DDDDDD	DDDDDD	DDDDDD	DDDDDD

Step 1 Calculate average percent wet (P) by adding up all wets and dividing by total number of observations.

$$\frac{\text{Total wet (w)} = 30}{\text{Total Observations} = 252} = .119$$

Step 2 Calculate warning limit with formula.

$$P + 2\sqrt{\frac{P\,(1 - p)}{N}}$$

When P = Average Percent wet
N = Number of subject in any 1 hour sample
(N in this case is 7)

$$.119 + 2\sqrt{\frac{.119\ (1 - .119)}{7}}$$

$$.119 + 2\sqrt{\frac{.119\ (.881)}{7}}$$

$$.119 + 2\sqrt{\frac{.105}{7}}$$

$.119 + 2\ .015$

$.119 + 2\ (.12)$

$.119 + .24 = .359$ or 36% Thus if 36% of the patients are wet, the sample is in the warning limit.

Step 3 Calculate the upper limit by the formula

$$P + 3\sqrt{\frac{\mathrm{P}\ (1 - \mathrm{p})}{\mathrm{N}}}$$

$$.119 + 3\sqrt{\frac{.119\ (.881)}{7}}$$

$.119 + 3\ \sqrt{.015}$

$.119 + 3\ (.12) =$

$.119 + .36 = .479$ or 48% Thus if 48% of the patients are wet in the sample mean, the upper limit has been reached.

QUALITY-CONTROL ASSESSMENT STANDARD DEVIATION OF VOLUMES—6-DAY ASSESSMENT PERIOD

Incontinence Volumes for Patient Smith	
	70
	50
	75
	125
	150
	100
	70
	115
	30
	50
	160
	150
	70
Total	1215

Formula

$$SD = \frac{\epsilon x^2 - \dfrac{(\epsilon \times 1^2)}{N}}{N - 1}$$

When $\epsilon \times {}^2$ = Sum of all squared volumes
$(\epsilon \times 1^2$ = square of the sum of all volumes
N = Total number of volume

Step 1 Add all volumes = 1215

Step 2 Calculate average by dividing number of step 1 by total number of volumes $\frac{1215}{13} = 93.4$

Step 3 Square all volumes and add the squared volumes
$70^2 + 50^2 + 75^2$ —— $+ 70^2 = 120{,}675$

Step 4 Square the sum in step 1 and divide this volume by the number of volumes that were added to obtain the sum.

$$\frac{(1215)^2}{13} = \frac{1476225}{13} = 113{,}555.76$$

Step 5 Subtract the volume obtained in step 3 from the sum in step 2
120,675 – 113,555.76 = 7120

Step 6 Divide the volume obtained in step 4 by $N - 1$ (In this example $N - 1 = 12$)

$$\frac{7120}{12} = 593.3$$

Step 7 Total the square root of Step 5 $\sqrt{593.3} = 24.3$

Step 8 Enter number in patient's control chart
Average expected wet = 93.4
Warning limit 93.4 + 2 Standard deviation above
93.4 + 2 (24.3) = 93.4 + 48.6 – 147.

TOILETING PATIENTS

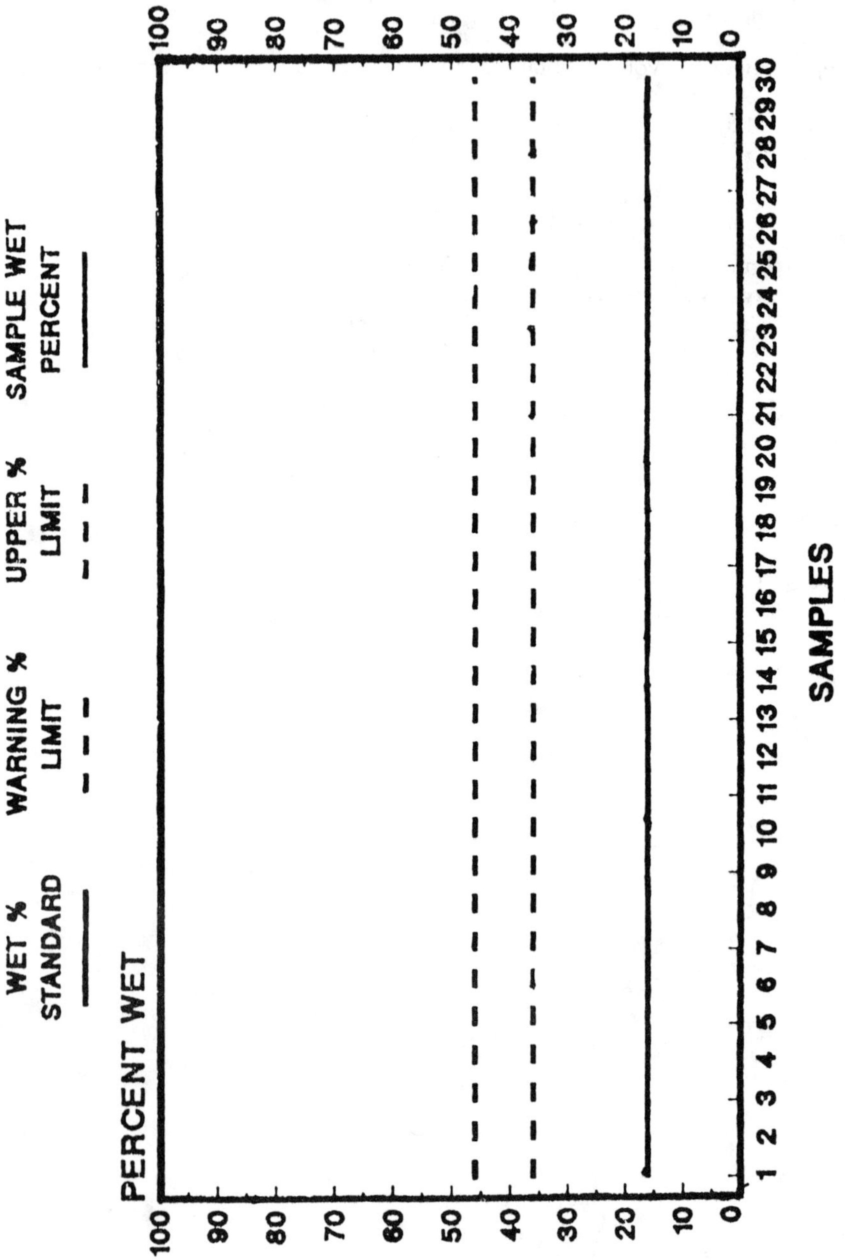

FINAL ASSESSMENT SUMMARY SHEET AND TREATMENT DECISION

Patient's Name ________________
Date ________________

Toileting Ability

Appropriate Toileting %	Check Appr. Box
0%–65% Poor ability to toilet	________
66%–75% Average ability to toilet	________
75%–100% Excellent ability to toilet	________

Bladder Storage Ability

Frequency of wets per day:

0–1 Good ability to prevent incontinence	________
1–2 Marginal ability to prevent incontinence	________
2+ Poor ability to prevent incontinence	________

Volume of wets per day:

0–30 cc Good ability to control urine loss	________
30–75 cc Marginal ability to control urine loss	________
75+ cc Poor ability to control urine loss	________

Mental Responsiveness

No question answered—poor responsiveness	________
Answered 50% correctly—marginal responsiveness	________
Answered 75% correctly—excellent responsiveness	________

6-Day Assessment Summary

Toileting ability

Column
1 total no. wets
2 total no. toilets
3 total no. voids (column 1 + 2)
4 percent appr. toilet $\frac{\text{(column 2)}}{\text{(column 3)}}$

Responsiveness

Column
8 no. yes correct responses
9 % correct $\frac{\text{(col. 8)}}{\text{\# days in prompted voiding} \times 6}$ =

Storage ability

5 No. expected wets per day $\frac{\text{(total wets)}}{6}$ =

6 Avg. vol. inc. episodes $\frac{\text{(add all inc. vols)}}{\text{(column 1)}}$ =

7 Lowest inc. vol ______
Largest Inc. vol ______

WETNESS VOLUME CONTROL CHART

Dry Weights of Pads

______ ______
______ ______

Patient name	Pad dry wgt.	Pad wet wgt.	Diff. wet vol.	Exp. wet	Warning wet	Checks in control out control	Patient position	Skin wet red OK

INDEX

INDEX